£16.99

WA292

Resuscitation in Primary Care

D1332933

Senior commissioning editor: Melanie Tait
Development editor: Zoë Youd
Production controller: Anthony Read
Desk editor: Claire Hutchins
Cover designer: Helen Brockway

Resuscitation in Primary Care

Michael Colquhoun BSc FRCP MRCGP DipIMC(RCS Ed)
General Practitioner, Malvern, UK
Honorary Secretary, Resuscitation Council (UK)

Philip Jevon BSc(Hons) RGN PGCE
Resuscitation Training Officer, Manor Hospital, Walsall, UK
Regional Representative, Resuscitation Council (UK)

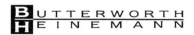

OXFORD AUCKLAND BOSTON JOHANNESBURG MELBOURNE NEW DELHI

Butterworth-Heinemann
An imprint of Elsevier Science Limited
Robert Stevenson House,
1–3 Baxter's Place, Leith Walk,
Edinburgh EH1 3AF

First published 2001
Reprinted 2002

British Library Cataloguing in Publication Data
A catalogue record for this book is available from the British Library

Library of Congress Cataloging in Publication Data
A catalog record for this book is available from the Library of Congress

ISBN 0 7506 4249 1

Typeset by Bath Typesetting
Printed and bound in Great Britain by MPG Books Ltd, Bodmin, Cornwall

Contents

Preface   vii

Acknowledgements   viii

Chapter 1 Cardiopulmonary arrest and the primary health care team   1

Chapter 2 Adult basic life support   9

Chapter 3 Adult advanced life support   23

Chapter 4 Management of the airway and ventilation   42

Chapter 5 Resuscitation in special circumstances   57

Chapter 6 Anaphylaxis   75

Chapter 7 Resuscitation of infants and children   82

Chapter 8 Resuscitation of the newly born   100

Chapter 9 Ethical and practical issues applied to resuscitation
          outside hospital   114

Chapter 10 Learning resuscitation techniques   123

Index   134

Preface

There can be few greater challenges to the skills of a health care provider than the resuscitation of a patient with cardiopulmonary arrest. This is particularly the case for those who work in the community where cardiac arrest (or other acute life-threatening emergencies) are usually unexpected and unpredictable. Any member of the primary health care team may, nevertheless, encounter such an emergency and will naturally be expected to know what to do.

Great advances have been made in our ability to resuscitate patients who collapse outside hospital in recent years. The recognition of the importance of early defibrillation and the development of the automated defibrillator have led to revolutionary changes in the ambulance service, and further technological advances have brought defibrillation within the scope of lay first aiders. At the same time, the appreciation of the importance of early basic life support provided by those who witness an arrest has led to a great increase in efforts to train the public in these techniques.

Members of the primary health care team will contribute to the resuscitation of many patients who collapse in the community either in their homes or occasionally at or near surgery premises. In other situations, prompt treatment of acutely ill patients may prevent cardiopulmonary arrest. In few other areas of medical practice will prompt correct treatment affect a patient's life so profoundly.

In this book we describe modern resuscitation methods and techniques with particular emphasis on their application in the community. Inevitably there is a bias towards the most frequent cause of cardiac arrest occurring outside of hospital — coronary heart disease — but we have also attempted to cover other important conditions that members of the primary health care team may encounter.

The procedures we recommend in this book all follow the guidelines of the European Resuscitation Council (endorsed by the Resuscitation Council (UK)); these have been publicized widely. These guidelines in turn are largely derived from recommendations made by the International Liaison Committee on Resuscitation, a body formed in 1992 with the aim of introducing guidelines for the practice of resuscitation applicable throughout the world.

This book is intended to provide practical guidance for members of the primary health care team, particularly general practitioners and nurses who work in the community. Hopefully other members of practice teams will find sections of interest and relevant to their role. We do not attempt to provide a comprehensive account of immediate medical care, rather our efforts are directed towards the everyday practitioner, practice and community nurses and other members of the primary health care team who will occasionally be confronted with patients with life-threatening conditions. We also hope that others who provide care for critically ill patients outside hospital, particularly ambulance personnel and first aiders, will also find information of interest.

M. C. Colquhoun
P. Jevon

Acknowledgements

We thank Keith Porter, David Drew and Jagtar Pooni for their invaluable comments and help with some sections of this book. We are grateful to the Resuscitation Council (UK) for permission to reproduce many diagrams and algorithms contained in their publications, particularly 'Resuscitation for the Citizen' and the '1998 Resuscitation Guidelines for use in the United Kingdom'. We thank John Hamilton and the Department of Medical Illustration at the Manor Hospital, Walsall for their invaluable help in producing many of the photographic illustrations. We are also grateful to Leo Bossaert of the European Resuscitation Council for their kind permission to reproduce CPR algorithms contained in their publication *European Resuscitation Council Guidelines for Resuscitation*. We also thank the following companies for permission to use their illustrations:

> Laerdal Medical (Orpington)
> Cook Critical Care
> Lifetec Medical

We thank the Terence Higgins Trust and King's College Hospital for permission to reproduce the standardized living will and for providing the most recent revision of this.

We thank our Secretaries Parmjit Cherra-Chapper and Lisa Fox, for the enormous amount of work they have carried out during the preparation of the manuscript; without their hard work the book would never have been published.

Chapter 1

Cardiopulmonary arrest and the primary health care team

Few medical emergencies challenge the skills of a medical professional to the same extent as the resuscitation of a patient with cardiopulmonary arrest. In this situation the ability of the personnel involved to deal with the situation may literally mean the difference between life and death for the patient.

The public, quite naturally, expect doctors, nurses and members of related professions to be able to deal with such emergencies, yet studies of resuscitation skills have consistently demonstrated major deficiencies in all groups of health care personnel tested. Surveys have also shown that many health care professionals who work in the community are inadequately equipped to resuscitate patients who collapse. This may be partly explained by the fact that patients with cardiopulmonary arrest are relatively unusual in everyday general practice, yet the evidence is clear that suitably trained practitioners equipped with defibrillators can resuscitate a substantial proportion of such patients.

Causes of cardiopulmonary arrest

Coronary heart disease is the commonest cause of sudden death encountered in the community, and cardiac arrest is particularly likely to occur in the early stages of myocardial infarction. About two-thirds of all patients who die of coronary disease do so outside hospital, around half in the first hour after the onset of symptoms, not because of serious heart muscle damage, but because ventricular fibrillation occurs. This lethal arrhythmia is a common complication of acute myocardial infarction and usually occurs before hospitalization and admission to the coronary care unit is possible. All practitioners who provide care for this vulnerable group of patients should be well equipped and trained to deal with the most common lethal complication of acute coronary syndromes; 5% of all patients with acute infarction attended by a general practitioner experience a cardiac arrest in his presence.

The primary care team may attempt to treat cardiopulmonary arrest due to many other causes, but numerically they are less important than coronary disease. Other cardiovascular disorders, including valve disease, cardiomyopathy and aneurysms, account for some cases as does cerebrovascular disease and subarachnoid haemorrhage. Trauma, electrocution, respiratory disease, near drowning, intoxication, hypovolaemia and drug overdosage may all lead to cardiopulmonary arrest outside hospital and therefore involve the primary health care team. Importantly, in many of these conditions cardiac arrest may be prevented by appropriate management (particularly of the airway) by someone trained in resuscitation skills.

Successful resuscitation – the chain of survival

For a patient to survive a cardiac arrest outside hospital, a sequence of separate events each need to take place and each of these can be likened to a link in a chain with each dependent on the others (Figure 1.1). Studies have consistently shown that survival is greatest when the arrest is witnessed by someone who can alert the emergency medical services so that help (and the defibrillator) are mobilized as soon as possible. Survival rates are highest when the rhythm is ventricular fibrillation, reflecting the relative difficulty of treating asystole and electromechanical dissociation (see below). When bystanders perform basic life support the chances of success are further increased, but the crucial determinant of survival is the time interval between collapse and defibrillation. The early availability of advanced life support techniques (which include advanced airway management skills, intravenous access and the use of drugs) further enhances the chance of survival. In communities with well-organized emergency medical services and a population well trained in basic life support, survival rates as high as 40% have been reported in patients receiving optimal treatment after cardiac arrest.

The chain of survival

For most members of the primary care team the first two links – calling for help and performing basic life support – are the most important. The final two links – defibrillation and advanced resuscitation techniques – have become widely available through the ambulance service during the last

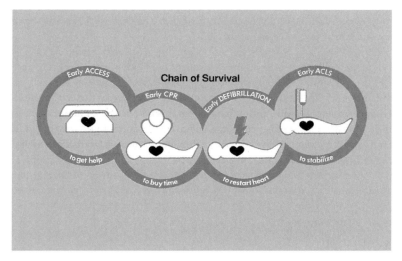

Figure 1.1 Chain of survival (Laerdal)

decade, but this should not detract from the advantages provided to a practice community when their doctors are also similarly equipped. The primary care team can then provide another level of skilled response for the victims of cardiopulmonary arrest.

Where a cardiac arrest is witnessed and a defibrillator is immediately available, defibrillation should be carried out as soon as possible. Survival rates in excess of 50% have been reported under these circumstances, both from the ambulance service and by general practitioners. This scenario is relatively common in cardiac arrests reported from primary care, particularly in patients in the early stages of myocardial infarction.

Practice organization

The response by the primary health care team to a patient who may need resuscitation must guarantee the attendance of appropriate personnel with suitable equipment. Much will depend on the particular circumstances, and will vary greatly in different practice areas; the response may also change at different times of the day. The importance of reaching the patient in the early stages of infarction as soon as possible has already been emphasized, and all practice staff, particularly receptionists who receive calls, must be aware of the significance of chest pain as a symptom of myocardial infarction. Practice policies should exist for such calls so that they are passed onto the doctor immediately.

Most current guidelines recommend that the ambulance service is summoned (on a 999 basis) to patients with chest pain, and a dual response by the general practitioner and the ambulance service has much to commend it. The ambulance service responds rapidly and is trained and equipped to resuscitate, while the general practitioner has diagnostic skills and may have relevant information about the patient's past history and medication. When a call is received that a patient has actually collapsed, the same dual response should be instigated.

Most practices have some arrangement whereby one or more partners are responsible for responding to urgent calls and reception staff must be able to contact the doctor with the minimum of delay by mobile phone, radio or message pager.

The equipment carried by an individual doctor will be determined by their level of expertise and the conditions under which they practise. When equipment (like a defibrillator) is shared among the doctors on call it is essential to have some foolproof method of handing the equipment over to the next doctor on duty. Although this sounds simple, it is not always straightforward when the duty doctor changes at weekends or over bank holidays.

Pathophysiology of cardiopulmonary arrest

There are three basic mechanisms of cardiac arrest – ventricular fibrillation, asystole and electromechanical dissociation. Pulseless ventricular tachycardia is an additional mode, but is usually classified with ventricular fibrillation because the causes and treatment are similar.

Ventricular fibrillation

Ventricular fibrillation is the commonest mode of cardiac arrest, particularly in patients with ischaemic heart disease, and is much more likely to respond to treatment than asystole or electromechanical dissociation. In patients with acute myocardial infarction who suffer a cardiac arrest, ventricular fibrillation (often preceded by ventricular tachycardia) is seen in around 90% of cases at the onset of the arrest; a similar figure has been reported in cardiac arrests witnessed by general practitioners.

The electrocardiogram shows a bizarre irregular waveform, apparently

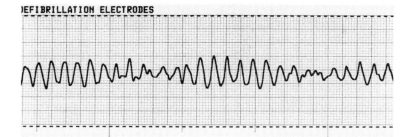

Figure 1.2 Ventricular fibrillation

random both in frequency and amplitude (Figure 1.2), reflecting the total loss of organized electrical activity in the myocardium. Ventricular fibrillation is an eminently treatable arrhythmia however, but the only effective treatment is defibrillation and the likelihood of success is crucially time dependent. Conditions for defibrillation are optimal for as little as 90 seconds after the onset of the rhythm, and the chances of success fall by about 10% with every minute that treatment is delayed. The major problem confronting all persons concerned with resuscitation is to minimize the time delay in providing the defibrillatory shock. Advances in defibrillator technology have greatly helped to simplify the technique by automating the process of rhythm recognition and the preparation to administer the shock. The training required to use a defibrillator is greatly reduced so that defibrillators are more widely available and capable of being used by a wider range of personnel. This is considered further in the chapter on advanced life support.

The amplitude of the ventricular fibrillation waveform becomes progressively finer with the passage of time until finally ending in asystole as myocardial oxygen and energy supplies are exhausted. Basic life support is a holding measure that 'buys time' until the defibrillator can be brought to the patient. It is effective because the relatively modest oxygenation and circulation provided prolongs the duration of ventricular fibrillation so that the patient is more likely to be in ventricular fibrillation when the defibrillator arrives.

Asystole

In asystolic cardiac arrest ventricular standstill is present because of the suppression of all natural cardiac pacemakers (Figure 1.3). Under normal circumstances failure of the normal sinus rhythm will lead to the appearance

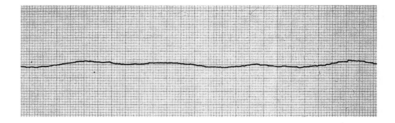

Figure 1.3 Asystole

of an escape rhythm maintained from a subsidiary pacemaker situated in the atrioventricular junction (junctional rhythm) or ventricular myocardium (idioventricular rhythm). Myocardial disease, hypoxia, drugs and electrolyte imbalance may all suppress this escape rhythm and cause asystole. Treatment of asystolic cardiac arrest is less commonly successful than when the rhythm is ventricular fibrillation but, nevertheless, patients do survive with appropriate treatment.

Untreated, ventricular fibrillation inevitably deteriorates into asystole as myocardial energy reserves and oxygen are exhausted and successful resuscitation at this late stage is almost impossible.

Electromechanical dissociation

The final mechanism producing cardiac arrest is electromechanical dissociation (EMD), a term used to signify the features of cardiac arrest associated with normal (or near normal) electrical excitation of the heart. The diagnosis is made on clinical grounds by the combination of the absence of a cardiac output with a rhythm on the monitor that would normally be accompanied by good ventricular function. The causes fall into two broad categories. In the first (sometimes called primary EMD) there is a failure of excitation contraction coupling in the cardiac myocytes resulting in profound loss of cardiac output. Causes include massive infarction, poisoning with drugs (beta blockers, calcium channel blockers) or toxins and electrolyte disturbance (hyperkalaemia, hypocalcaemia). In secondary EMD there is a mechanical barrier to ventricular filling or ejection. Causes include cardiac tamponade or rupture, tension pneumothorax, pulmonary embolism, occlusion of prosthetic heart valves and hypovolaemia. In all cases treatment is directed towards the cause.

Resuscitation training

Although members of the primary health care team may be called on to resuscitate a patient relatively infrequently, they must, nevertheless, be trained and equipped to provide a level of care appropriate to their role.

Basic life saving skills should be possessed by all personnel who come into contact with patients yet, in reality, the skills are often not well taught, practised or updated. This is particularly the situation in primary care where such serious emergencies occur relatively infrequently, and many members of the primary health care team may not feel the incentive to learn or practise emergency life support skills.

Resuscitation techniques may be conveniently divided into different levels of attainment, which have implications for the training of staff. Basic life support means the provision of respiration and the maintenance of the circulation without the use of special equipment. In practice this means the assessment of the casualty, the provision of rescue breathing to provide oxygenation and chest compressions to provide a circulation. The use of simple barrier devices that do not pass the oropharynx (faceshields and masks) is often included in this definition. Without the provision of effective basic life support, few victims of sudden death will benefit from more advanced life saving techniques like defibrillation.

The term 'basic life support with airway adjuncts' describes the practice of basic life support with special equipment designed to assist the maintenance of the airway and provision of respiration. Facemasks, with or without self-inflating bags, would be included as would simple airway devices like the Guedal airway.

Basic life support techniques should be taught to all the population, and experience from Europe and certain areas of the USA testifies to the value of this. The care of the airway, especially in an unconscious casualty may be life saving, and the provision of expired air ventilation alone may save the victim of near drowning. All members of the practice team should be taught the techniques and practice them on training manikins. The use of airway adjuncts might be included, especially for the nursing members of the team.

The Royal College of General Practitioners has recognized the importance of basic life support by insisting that all prospective candidates for its membership examination have demonstrated competence in the techniques.

The term 'advanced life support (ALS)' describes the skills necessary to manage a patient with cardiopulmonary arrest, and includes more advanced airway techniques (endotracheal intubation and the use of the laryngeal mask) as well as defibrillation and the use of drugs. The ambulance service in the UK are now well equipped to provide advanced life support to victims who collapse in the community, and members of the primary health care team may find themselves working with them. Many general practitioners learn and practise ALS techniques during their hospital experience, but regular practice and updating is required to maintain competency.

Increasingly, the divisions within these categories are becoming less distinct. Modern 'smart' defibrillators have automated the process of cardiac rhythm recognition and delivery of a defibrillatory shock enabling their use by a wide range of personnel; practice nurses and reception staff could learn to use them relatively easily.

Sources of training

Most health districts now have a resuscitation training officer who coordinates training in resuscitation techniques (especially advanced techniques) in their area. Many assist in training members of the primary health care team and organize special sessions for this purpose, and can be contacted through the hospital switchboard.

Training in basic life support may also be arranged through the voluntary aid societies (St John Ambulance, the British Red Cross and St Andrew's Ambulance Association in Scotland) or the Royal Life Saving Society, who run courses in first aid or water rescue. Heartstart UK is a national campaign coordinated by the British Heart Foundation that teaches emergency life support skills in a single session and many of the groups offer training in basic life support to practice staff in their locality.

The advanced life support course administered by the Resuscitation Council UK is an intensive course, usually lasting 2 days, during which comprehensive instruction in advanced life support is combined with practical experience. The course combines standardized lectures and skill stations in which techniques are taught in a uniform way to an agreed standard regardless of where the course is held. Candidates are taught by instructors who have completed an instructors' course in which the techniques of adult education are stressed. Although primarily intended for hospital staff, many general practitioners have successfully completed the course. More details about these and related courses are provided in Chapter 9.

Chapter 2

Adult basic life support

The term 'basic life support' is used to describe the maintenance of breathing and the circulation without special equipment. The use of airway adjuncts that do not pass the oropharynx (like protective shields and facemasks) is usually included in the term. For the great majority of adult victims of cardiopulmonary arrest, basic life support is merely a holding procedure, buying time until more advanced procedures, especially defibrillation, are available. Although basic life support by itself will not restore a spontaneous circulation in a patient who has suffered a cardiac arrest, the techniques may be all that is required where the problem is primarily respiratory, for example in the case of near drowning.

Considerable effort has been devoted to training members of the lay population to perform basic life support in recent years. Studies in many countries have shown unequivocally that the prompt institution of cardiopulmonary resuscitation, or CPR, by a bystander who witnesses a cardiac arrest improves the outcome considerably. In the UK, basic life support is taught as part of first aid courses run by the voluntary aid societies or as part of the water rescue classes of the Royal Life Saving Society. Recent years have seen an expansion of small local schemes dedicated to teaching basic life support in a single class lasting about 2 hours. The first of these was established in Brighton more than 20 years ago and there are now several hundred schemes coordinated by the British Heart Foundation as part of its 'Heartstart UK' initiative. Although CPR is mentioned in the national curriculum, it is not a compulsory subject, and the teaching of CPR in schools remains patchy and dependent upon the enthusiasm of individual teachers.

The ability to perform basic life support competently should be a mandatory requirement of all health care professionals, yet many studies have demonstrated serious shortcomings in their ability to do so. Teaching of hospital staff has become more widespread and standardized with the widespread appointment of Resuscitation Training Officers, but training for personnel who work in the community is not so well established; no formal

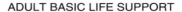

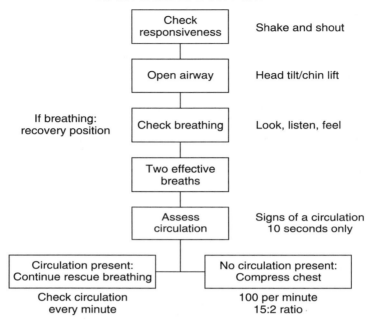

Send or go for help as soon as possible according to guidelines

Figure 2.1 European Resuscitation Council Guidelines for Basic Life Support
©ERC 1999 (from *European Resuscitation Council Guidelines for Resuscitation*,
edited by L. Bossaert, 1998, Elsevier, Oxford by kind permission)

mechanism exists in many health districts. CPR is essentially a practical skill
and training on manikins is necessary to acquire expertise. Skill decay after
training occurs rapidly and frequent refresher classes with manikin practice
are needed to maintain expertise. The logistics of providing satisfactory
training for members of the practice team are formidable, yet not
insuperable, especially when the help of the local Resuscitation Training
Officer or Ambulance Training School can be enlisted.

For over 10 years the Royal College of General Practitioners has required
candidates for their membership examination to demonstrate proficiency in
basic life support. There have been no formal studies of the effect of this
policy, but one study that tested the ability of general practitioners to
perform basic life support (many of who were members of the College)
demonstrated severe deficiencies in their abilities.

Procedures for the performance of basic life support

The procedures described here and the sequence in which they are carried out (Figure 2.1) are based on the recommendations of the International Liaison Committee on Resuscitation (ILCOR, 1997) and endorsed by the European Resuscitation Council in 1998. They have been adopted as standard practice throughout the UK, Europe and many other countries of the world.

The performance of basic life support involves the assessment of the casualty with subsequent steps determined by the findings. The widely used mnemonic 'ABC' is commonly applied – A stands for assessment and airway, B for breathing and C for circulation.

A – Assessment

- The first stage of the assessment should be a quick check for any dangers to the casualty or the rescuer. Hazards like gas, toxins, electricity, fire or traffic are usually self-evident.
- Check responsiveness. Shake the victim gently by the shoulders but be careful not to aggravate any existing injury, particularly of the cervical spine. Also call out the victim's name if it is known. If there is no response shout for help.

B – Breathing

The neck should be extended to lift the tongue off the posterior wall of the pharynx. The recommended method is the head tilt, chin lift technique where one hand is placed on the forehead of the victim and used to exert pressure to tilt the head backwards. At the same time two fingers of the other hand are placed under the point of the chin to lift it forward; this should lift the tongue clear of the posterior pharyngeal wall and establish a patent airway (Figure 2.2). Having done this look, listen and feel for evidence of breathing.

- Look for chest movement.
- Listen near the mouth and nose for breath sounds.
- Feel for ventilation against your cheek (Figure 2.3). Ten seconds should be allowed for this before deciding that breathing is absent.

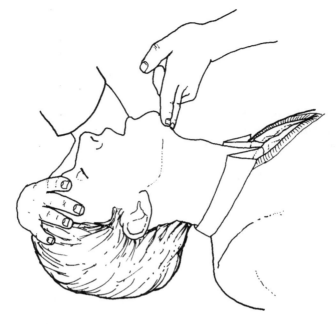

Figure 2.2 Head tilt, chin lift

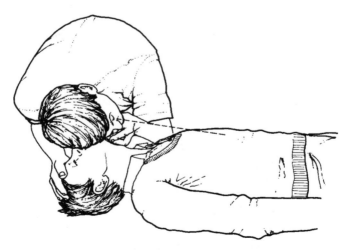

Figure 2.3 Look, listen and feel for evidence of breathing

If the casualty is unconscious but *breathing adequately*, place him or her in the recovery position. The most recent ILCOR guidelines do not recommend one specific recovery position – intense debate continues about the relative merits of a number of recovery positions that have been described. The important points about the position adopted should be that the casualty is in a stable, safe posture in as near a lateral position as possible with the head dependent to allow free drainage of fluids. Any pressure on the chest that impairs breathing should be avoided. It should be possible to monitor the casualty's breathing and gain access to the airway should it be required. It should also be possible to turn the victim onto the side or the back easily and safely, having due regard to the possibility of cervical spine injury. At this stage the emergency services must be summoned (if this has not being done already).

If a casualty is *not breathing* send another person to summon an ambulance, but if you are on your own do this yourself. If the victim is a child or the victim of near drowning or trauma, however, the likelihood is that you are dealing primarily with a respiratory arrest and resuscitation should be applied for one minute before summoning help.

A patent airway should be maintained by the head tilt, chin lift method already described. Any obvious obstruction in the mouth should be removed, but well fitting dentures are best left in place. The traditional method of ventilating the casualty by expired air ventilation employs the

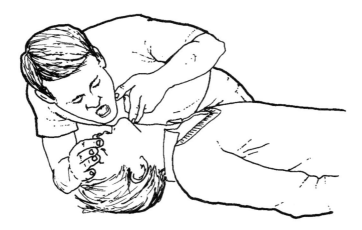

Figure 2.4 Maintain head tilt chin lift, pinch the nose, take a deep breath in and place your mouth completely over the casualty's mouth ensuring a good seal

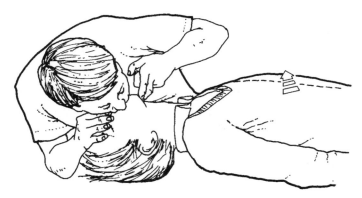

Figure 2.5 Breathe slowly into the casualty until the chest is seen to rise

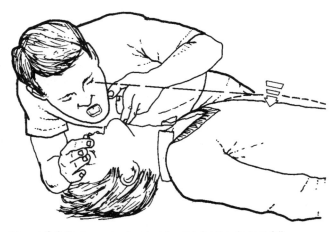

Figure 2.6 Remove your head and watch for the chest to fall

mouth-to-mouth method. The nose is pinched closed with the thumb and forefinger of the hand already placed on the forehead and the rescuer's lips are firmly sealed round those of the victim (Figure 2.4). The rescuer breathes into the casualty until the chest is seen to rise, taking about one and one half seconds to inflate the chest (Figure 2.5). The rescuer then removes his or her head and the victim's chest will fall (Figure 2.6). The process is then repeated. Each breath should visibly expand the chest, but it is important not to over-inflate the chest and cause air to enter the oesophagus and stomach with resultant gastric distension. This increases

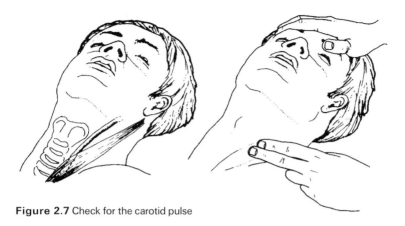

Figure 2.7 Check for the carotid pulse

the risk of vomiting or regurgitation with the danger of pulmonary aspiration. After two rescue breaths have been successfully performed (or after five attempts if unsuccessful), if breathing is still absent check for signs of a circulation.

In the context of basic life support performed by professional health care workers, a barrier device or facemask should be available and it should not normally be necessary to perform mouth-to-mouth artificial respiration on patients. A number of barrier devices are available and most feature a plastic sheet with a valve or similar devices to permit ventilation without allowing the return of secretions from the victim. Whichever device is chosen, staff must know where to find it and be well practised in its use.

In the authors' view far the best device for use in primary care is the Laerdal pocket mask. This resembles the anaesthetist's mask and fits snugly over the mouth and nose of the casualty to provide an airtight seal (see Figure 2.12). Ventilation is provided through an aperture to which a one-way valve can be fitted. The device is also compatible with most self-inflating bags. It is inexpensive and should be carried in the general practitioner's case and should be available in all consulting rooms, treatment areas and in reception.

C – Circulation

Taking no longer than ten seconds, assess the casualty for signs of a circulation. Check for the presence of a pulse – the best artery is the carotid (Figure 2.7), but the femoral is an acceptable alternative. Also look for other

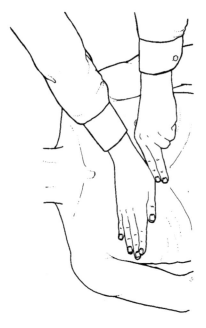

Figure 2.8 Locate the xiphisternum, place the middle finger on this point, and the index finger on the bony sternum just above. Slide the heel of the other hand down to meet them

signs of a circulation including swallowing, movement and breathing (more than an occasional gasp).

If there are signs of a circulation, continue with rescue breathing but re-check the circulation after every ten breaths or approximately every minute. If the casualty starts to breathe but remains unresponsive, place in the recovery position and observe closely.

If there are no signs of a circulation chest compressions should be performed without delay. Ensure that the casualty is on their back on a firm flat surface.

- The correct place to compress the chest is in the centre of the lower half of the sternum. To locate this position, use the index and middle fingers to identify the lower rib margins and slide the fingers up to the xiphisternum. Place the middle finger on this point and position the index finger on the bony sternum just above. Slide the heel of your other hand down to meet the fingers and leave the heel of the hand in this position (Figure 2.8). Remove the first hand and place it on top of

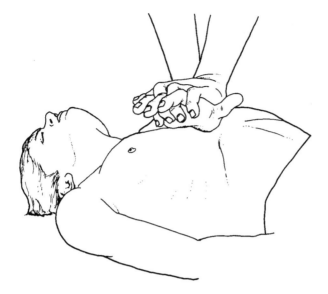

Figure 2.9 Remove the first hand, place it on top of the second and interlock the fingers

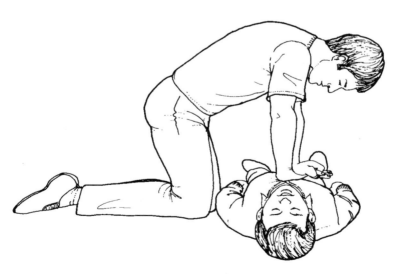

Figure 2.10 Compress the sternum firmly with the hands straight and the elbows locked with your shoulders positioned vertically above the casualty's sternum

the second, interlocking the fingers and lifting them up to ensure that pressure is not exerted on the costal cartilages (Figure 2.9).

- Compress the sternum firmly with the arms straight and the elbows locked with your shoulders positioned vertically above the casualty's sternum (Figure 2.10). Compress the sternum approximately 4–5 cm aiming for a rate of about 100 compressions a minute, i.e. just under two per second. Approximately the same time should be spent in the compression phase as in the relaxation phase of the cycle. After every 15 compressions give a further two breaths, returning your hands immediately to the sternum to administer a further 15 compressions. The ratio of 15 compressions to two breaths should be maintained without further pulse checks or pauses unless the casualty attempts to breathe or shows signs of a spontaneous circulation.

Two rescuer CPR

If two persons trained in the techniques of basic life support are available, one should perform rescue breathing while the other should assume responsibility for chest compressions. The compression rate should again be 100 per minute and the 1998 guidelines recommend a ratio of five compressions to one ventilation with a pause after the fifth compression long enough to allow a breath to be given over 1½–2 seconds. Provided the airway is maintained in the open position, it is not necessary to wait for the chest to deflate before resuming chest compressions.

Recent experimental studies have shown that the coronary perfusion pressure rises progressively during a sequence of chest compressions and falls rapidly when the compressions cease during ventilation. More than five compressions are required to achieve maximal coronary perfusion, and a longer series of compressions enables this to be achieved and maintained for a longer period of time. Future guidelines are likely to recommend that a ratio of 15 compressions to 2 ventilations is also employed in two rescuer CPR.

Choking

It is extremely rare for members of the primary health care team to attempt the treatment of a previously healthy individual who is choking. It is important to be aware of the recommended techniques, however, because parents often ask about the treatment of choking children and occasionally carers of patients with swallowing difficulties ask about the correct techniques to be adopted.

If the casualty is breathing he or she should be encouraged to cough, but if airway obstruction appears to be complete, attempt to remove a foreign body by finger sweeps in the mouth. If this is unsuccessful administer five back blows to the area between the scapulae.

- Lean the casualty forward to encourage any dislodged foreign body to be ejected rather than move further down the airway.
- While supporting the casualty's chest with one hand, use the heel of the other hand to deliver up to five back slaps between the scapulae. If the casualty is lying down or is unconscious roll him or her towards you supporting the chest with your thighs and deliver up to five back blows between the scapulae.

If back blows are not successful abdominal thrusts should be performed (the Heimlich manoeuvre). Standing behind the casualty, make a fist with one hand and place it immediately below the xiphisternum. Grasp this fist with your other hand and push firmly and rapidly upwards and posteriorly towards the casualty's spine, i.e. towards yourself.

If the casualty is lying down, kneel astride the victim placed in the supine position. Position the heel of the hand above the umbilicus but below the xiphoid process. The other hand should be placed on top of this and abdominal thrusts should be administered by pressing firmly downwards and superiorly towards the victim's chest. If abdominal thrusts are unsuccessful, it is recommended that further back blows are administered. The treatment of choking in children is described in the chapter on paediatric resuscitation. Recent studies have shown that conventional chest compressions create higher pressures in the airway than abdominal thrusts, and furture guidelines are likely to recommend chest compressions in the unconscious choking adult instead of the procedures recommended above.

Precordial thump

A precordial thump is recommended in cases of monitored or witnessed cardiac arrest and is therefore more properly considered an advanced life support technique. It would be appropriate for many health care providers to use the technique and there are anecdote accounts of its successful use by GPs. It is important that it is performed correctly. The blow should be

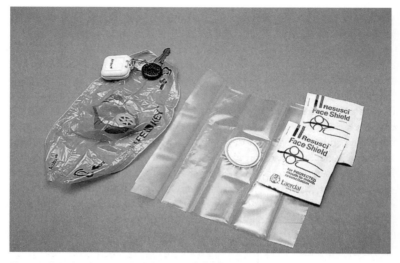

Figure 2.11 Barrier devices: The Life Key and a Face Shield

delivered to the area of the chest at the lower left sternum overlying the heart. A sharp blow should be delivered with the medial side of the fist which is then rapidly withdrawn from the chest wall. A precordial thump is unlikely to be successful after ventricular fibrillation (or pulseless ventricular tachycardia) has been present for more than 30 seconds.

Risks to the rescuer

The possibility of the transmission of infection from a patient to the rescuer has been the subject of much concern recently, heightened by fears of the transmission of hepatitis B and the human immune deficiency virus (HIV), both diseases with a high mortality rate. No case of the acquired immune deficiency syndrome (AIDS) or hepatitis B has yet been reported, however, in a rescuer as a result of performing mouth-to-mouth ventilation. Although the HIV virus is present in saliva it does not seem that transmission occurs via this route in the absence of blood-to-blood contact. All health care workers who come into contact with patients in the UK should now be immunized against hepatitis B.

There have, however, been a small number of reports of the transmission of other infections to a rescuer following mouth-to-mouth resuscitation. These include meningococcal disease, tuberculosis, herpes simplex and salmonella. Such cases are extremely rare and the barrier devices available should provide adequate protection.

Many people will feel the need for some form of protective barrier device (Figure 2.11), particularly if saliva is contaminated with blood, as may occur in the context of trauma. Any such device must function effectively in both its protective role and permit effective ventilation. There should be adequate training in the use of the device which should not hinder the flow of air or provide too great a dead space. Even more importantly, the equipment must be immediately available whenever it is required. In the authors' view the most suitable equipment for use in primary care is the Laerdal pocket mask (Figure 2.12).

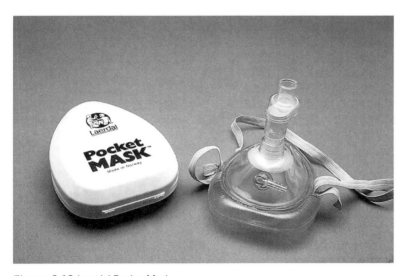

Figure 2.12 Laerdal Pocket Mask

There is a small risk of infection following needlestick injuries. Great care should be taken with the use of needles and intravenous cannulae which must be disposed of properly in a suitable container. If a needlestick injury does occur the protocol recommended by the local Department of Occupational Health should be followed in all cases.

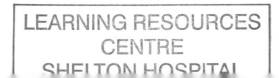

Active compression/decompression CPR

This technique of performing chest compression was developed after an isolated case report from San Francisco where a patient was successfully resuscitated when the rescuer performed chest compressions with a plumber's plunger placed on the chest wall. The circumstances of this resuscitation were such that it seemed that this novel method of performing CPR may have contributed to the victim's survival. It was suggested that the negative pressure applied to the thorax when the plunger was lifted up might improve venous return (and hence cardiac output) and also assist ventilation. A commercial device is available. This features a suction cup which is applied to the skin of the chest over the lower sternum. It is used to compress the chest, and after each compression it is lifted up – the suction cup remaining in contact with the skin – to decompress the thorax. Experimental studies have shown improved cardiac output and coronary perfusion with the use of this device but, unfortunately, most clinical trials have not shown an improvement in outcome, and there is a significant risk of causing injury to the casualty. At present it cannot be recommended for pre-hospital use.

References and further reading

Handley AJ, Becker LB, Allen M *et al.* (1997) An advisory statement from the Basic Life Support Working Group of the International Liaison Committee on Resuscitation (ILCOR). *Resuscitation*, **34**:101–8.

Handley AJ, Bahr J, Basket P *et al.* (1998) The 1998 European Resuscitation guidelines for adult single rescuer basic life support. *Resuscitation*, **37**:67–80.

Handley AJ (1999) Basic life support. In: *ABC of Resuscitation*, 4th edn (Colquhoun MC, Handley AJ, Evans TR, eds). BMJ Publishing Group, London.

Nolan J, Gwinnett C (1998) The 1998 European Resuscitation Council guidelines for adult single rescuer basic life support. *BMJ*, **316**:1870–6.

Zideman DA (1999) Aids, Hepatitis and Resuscitation. In: *ABC of Resuscitation*, 4th edn (Colquhoun MC, Handley AJ, Evans TR, eds). pp 52–3. BMJ Publishing Group, London

Chapter 3

Adult advanced life support

The term 'advanced life support' is used to describe the more specialized techniques used to maintain breathing and the circulation during resuscitation attempts, as well as the actual methods of treatment employed to try to restore the cardiac output of patients who have suffered cardiopulmonary arrest. The majority of patients who are successfully resuscitated are those in ventricular fibrillation. This is the most common mode of cardiac arrest in patients with coronary disease and accounts for the majority of patients likely to require resuscitation by members of the primary health care team. The single most important advanced life support technique therefore is defibrillation, and this has been made considerably easier in recent years, largely due to advances in defibrillator technology. Defibrillators are now cheaper and more widely available and capable of being used by the lay public let alone health care professionals. If there is one advanced life support technique that should be known by general practitioners it is defibrillation because this will do more good for more patients than any other.

Defibrillators and defibrillation

The defibrillator is a device designed to administer an electrical counter-shock to the heart that is fibrillating. The shock aims to depolarize a critical mass of the myocardium to interrupt the fibrillation wavefront and allow the natural pacemaking tissue to resume control of the heart with the return of an organized rhythm and cardiac output. A precordial thump may abolish the arrhythmia when applied very soon after the onset of ventricular fibrillation and should be considered in cases of witnessed — especially monitored — cardiac arrest.

Electrical energy from batteries or from the mains is used to charge a capacitor, and the stored energy is subsequently discharged through electrodes placed on the victim's chest wall. The objective is to achieve the

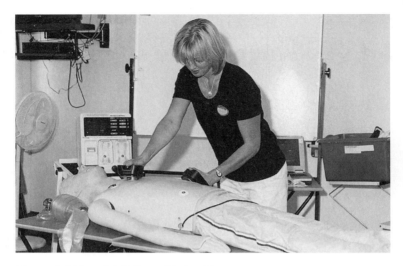

Figure 3.1 Manual defibrillator (Medtronic)

maximum current flow through the heart, and this is measured as the energy delivered from the device in joules (J), the usual energies employed being 200 J and 360 J.

Modern defibrillators monitor the electrocardiogram through the same electrodes that are used to deliver the shock. With the traditional manual defibrillator (Figure 3.1) the operator interprets the rhythm displayed on the monitor screen and decides whether a shock is indicated. The energy of the shock is selected manually, the capacitor is charged, and the shock is given without removing the electrodes from the chest wall; most modern manual defibrillators incorporate controls in the handles of the electrodes to facilitate this procedure. Considerable skill, training and experience are necessary to use this type of defibrillator safely and effectively, largely because of the need to interpret the electrocardiogram.

Automated defibrillators

A quantum leap in the practice of defibrillation occurred with the advent of the semiautomatic advisory defibrillator (Figure 3.2). This machine abolished the need for the operator to interpret the electrocardiogram, decide if a shock was required and charge the machine to the appropriate energy level. With the semiautomatic defibrillator these tasks are performed

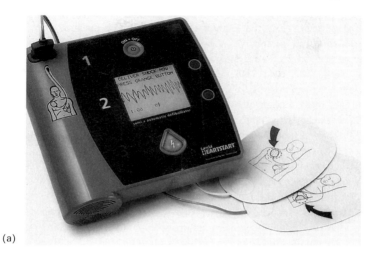

(a)

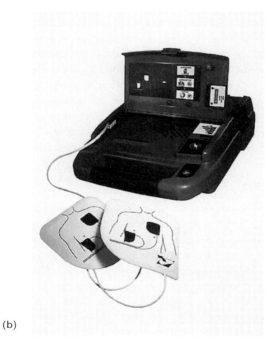

(b)

Figure 3.2 (a) The Forerunner (Laerdal) and (b) The First Save (Lifetec)

automatically by electronic circuitry contained in the machine. The main requirement of the operator is to decide that cardiac arrest may have occurred and attach two adhesive electrodes to the patient's chest wall. These serve the dual role of monitoring the electrocardiogram and delivering the countershock. Instructions are provided on a liquid crystal screen and most models also incorporate a synthesized voice which gives audible commands to reinforce these.

While the machine is interpreting the electrocardiogram the patient must be as still as possible and basic life support must cease. This process takes 10 seconds or less and if a rhythm likely to respond to a countershock is detected (ventricular fibrillation or ventricular tachycardia above a predetermined rate), the machine charges itself to the appropriate energy level and indicates to the operator that a shock is indicated. A pass card or manual override facility is usually incorporated so that the machine may be used as a manual defibrillator if more highly trained staff arrive at the scene. The machine is capable of sophisticated data collection for later playback and analysis as part of audit or training.

It was the advisory defibrillator (often known as the automated external defibrillator or AED) that enabled the introduction of defibrillators to be achieved so rapidly throughout the ambulance service in the UK, and Scotland became the first country in the world to equip every emergency ambulance with a defibrillator. The simplicity of operation greatly reduced the training requirements needed to perform defibrillation and less highly trained grades of staff than the paramedic were soon able to use the automated defibrillator. Published evidence subsequently testified to the effectiveness of defibrillation performed by ambulance technicians.

First responder defibrillators

The simplicity of use and the effectiveness of automated defibrillators have been extended with the 'first responder' defibrillator. This is an automated defibrillator principally designed for use by people without extensive training, including first aiders and other members of the general public, who may only perform the procedure infrequently. The machines are designed for long periods of storage before use with minimal maintenance and have simplicity of operation as a key design feature. Controls are reduced to a minimum and most models do not have the ECG monitor screens or manual override facilities required by more highly trained personnel. Clear instructions are provided on a screen or by voice prompts. The machines are quite sophisticated in fact, and are able to store considerable amounts of data recorded during use. They also perform automatic checks on battery status during prolonged periods between use and indicate when servicing or battery replacement is required.

The price of first responder defibrillators is considerably less than the cost of a conventional manual or automated defibrillator and they have proved very attractive to those who need to be equipped to defibrillate effectively yet only do it infrequently. The voluntary aid societies have equipped their first aiders who attend public duties with these machines, and there are several reports of their successful use. They are lightweight, compact, portable and require very little maintenance; they are ideally suited for use in general practice.

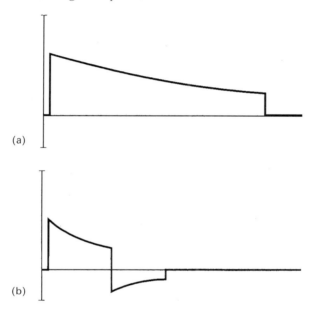

Figure 3.3 (a) Monophasic and (b) biphasic waveforms (from The First Save Star Technology, Optimised Current Delivery for Successful Defibrillation, S. Hildage, by kind permission)

Biphasic defibrillators

Experimental work undertaken during the development of the implantable defibrillator has shown that the characteristics of the defibrillatory shock may greatly influence its efficacy in terminating ventricular fibrillation. The output waveform of the conventional defibrillator follows a monophasic sinusoidal pattern, and this has been shown to be less efficient than a biphasic shock where the polarity of the waveform is reversed during the shock (Figure 3.3a and b). External defibrillators that utilize the biphasic waveform have been extensively investigated in humans during the testing of implanted defibrillators and have been shown consistently to be more efficient than monophasic ones. The practical significance is that lower energy shocks may be used with biphasic defibrillators with less risk of damage to the myocardium. The lower energy requirement has major implications for defibrillator design as smaller batteries and capacitors may be used, electronic switching within the machine is simplified and other components may be made more compact; the machines are therefore smaller and lighter. External defibrillators that employ biphasic shocks are now available commercially and likely to become the standard in the future. The potential advantages of this technology have been particularly exploited by the makers of the first responder defibrillator to reduce the size and weight of the machines while hopefully offering an advantage in clinical use, although this has not been established conclusively in clinical trials at the time of writing.

The management of cardiac arrest – the universal algorithm

The most recent advanced life support guidelines published by the European Resuscitation Council (ERC) are based on the advisory statements of the International Liaison Committee on Resuscitation (ILCOR) which were produced in 1997 and adopted for use in the UK in the same year. Their adoption throughout Europe in 1998 marked a major landmark in international cooperation in the production of resuscitation guidelines. The procedures described in this chapter for the management of adult cardiac arrest are based on the recommendations contained in the ERC guidelines which are endorsed for use in the UK by the Resuscitation Council UK.

The advent of the automated external defibrillator (AED) was one major reason for the requirement to update the previous 1992 guidelines, which had required the operator to interpret the cardiac rhythm and make decisions in the light of the ECG rhythm recognized. AEDs interpret the rhythm automatically and the 1998 guidelines are designed to be equally applicable to manual or automated external defibrillators. Decision-making

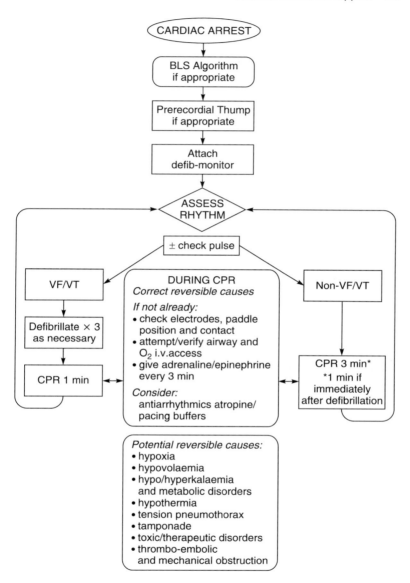

Figure 3.4 European Resuscitation Council Guidelines for Advanced Life Support ©ERC 1999 (from *European Resuscitation Council Guidelines for Resuscitation,* edited by L. Bossaert, 1998, Elsevier, Oxford by kind permission)

has been reduced to a minimum to simplify operation whenever possible, while allowing those with more extensive knowledge to apply their skills.

The ERC guideline document stresses that there are limitations to guidelines, and that they must be applied with common sense and an appreciation of their intent. Interpretation may vary with the environment in which they are employed, and specific modifications to the procedures recommended may be required in cases of trauma, hypothermia, drug overdosage, anaphylaxis and pregnancy.

The approach to the resuscitation of adult victims of cardiac arrest is illustrated in the universal algorithm shown in Figure 3.4. It is inherent in the application of this algorithm that the successive steps are only undertaken if the preceding one has been unsuccessful. Entry into the algorithm depends on the circumstances surrounding the arrest. If basic life support is in progress it should continue while the defibrillator/monitor is attached. For patients that are already monitored the ECG and clinical detection of cardiac arrest should be almost simultaneous. A precordial thump may abolish ventricular tachyarrhythmias and should be considered in cases of witnessed cardiac arrest, especially if there is likely to be any delay in monitoring the rhythm.

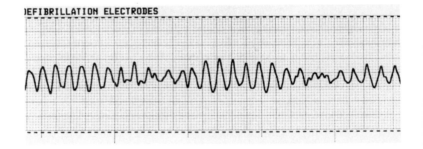

Figure 3.5 Ventricular fibrillation

The cardiac rhythm is the key determinant of the procedures to be followed and, depending on the rhythm detected, the algorithm is followed in one of two ways based on whether the rhythm is ventricular fibrillation/pulseless ventricular tachycardia (which will be interpreted as a shockable rhythm in the case of an AED) (Figure 3.5) or other rhythms (when an AED will state that no shock is indicated).

Ventricular fibrillation/tachycardia

Defibrillatory shocks are administered in groups of three; the first shock should be given with the minimum of delay at a delivered energy of 200 J. If this is unsuccessful it should be repeated once at the same energy level. This may succeed when a previous shock at the same energy has been unsuccessful because successful defibrillation depends on many variables that change from moment to moment. In particular, transthoracic impedance may be reduced by the first shock allowing more favourable conditions for the second. There is no evidence that initial shocks at a higher energy level are more likely to be successful and they risk greater damage to the myocardium.

If the second shock is unsuccessful the third shock is given at 360 J. The energy level is selected from a dial or some similar arrangement with manual defibrillators while it is increased automatically with automated defibrillators. Subsequent shocks should all be at 360 J unless a coordinated rhythm is re-established and a further cardiac arrest occurs; shocks at 200 J may be given initially in this situation.

Defibrillators that employ a biphasic shock waveform will deliver shocks of lower energy but with equivalent efficacy to those of the standard energy levels given as a monophasic shock.

A pulse check should be carried out (and will be prompted by an AED) if the rhythm changes to one compatible with a cardiac output. Modern defibrillators usually charge rapidly and it should be possible to deliver the set of three shocks within 30–45 seconds and the sequence should not be interrupted by basic life support. If it is not possible to deliver the shocks rapidly (because of inexperience or the use of old equipment), a few cycles of basic life support may be given between shocks.

After a shock is given the ECG monitor screen will often show a straight line or be distorted by artefact; this does not necessarily mean that asystole has resulted and it may be some seconds before a trace of diagnostic quality is produced. This may ultimately demonstrate that a coordinated rhythm has been restored or that the original rhythm persists. If the monitor screen of a manual defibrillator shows a straight line for more than one sweep of the screen after the shock, 1 minute of CPR should be given (without a dose of adrenaline) before the rhythm is reassessed.

Over 80% of those successfully resuscitated will be defibrillated by one of the first three shocks. If these fail, the best prospects for restoring a perfusing rhythm still lie with defibrillation but, at this point, the priority changes to the provision of basic life support to preserve cerebral function and, if possible, delay further myocardial deterioration. One minute of CPR should be given at this stage before attempting further defibrillation. Ideally, adrenaline is given before the second set of shocks (and with each subsequent loop of the algorithm) to enhance the efficiency of basic life support if intravenous or endotracheal access has been secured. During CPR attempts can be made (if help is available) to institute advanced airway management procedures and gain intravenous access to allow the administration of drugs. It should be obvious that there are great advantages for any member of the primary health care team to be working with the ambulance service when attempting to resuscitate a patient.

A search for potentially reversible causes or aggravating factors should be made at this point and corrected if identified. Possible causes include electrolyte imbalance, hypothermia and drug overdose or toxicity for which specific treatment may be indicated. The management of many of these will pose a major problem outside hospital, especially if working with limited assistance.

If none of the second set of shocks is successful, the loop indicated in the left-hand side of the algorithm is repeated. Each cycle of the loop provides a further chance (while CPR is being undertaken) for attempts at intubation or venous cannulation, administration of adrenaline and consideration of the use of antiarrhythmic or buffering agents. The ERC guidelines suggest that antiarrhythmic drugs may be considered in the presence of persistent ventricular fibrillation or tachycardia resistant to countershock after two to four loops of the algorithm (i.e. 6–12 shocks). No convincing evidence exists for their effectiveness in this desperate situation and no specific agents are recommended. Lignocaine, amiodarone and bretylium have been advocated, and trials are currently in progress to define their role more precisely. It is unlikely that these agents will be available in primary care, and there is insufficient evidence available at present to recommend that they should be.

Technique of defibrillation

Correct technique is important during defibrillation. AEDs utilize adhesive electrodes incorporating coupling gel to ensure good electrical contact with the chest wall, but care is needed with manual defibrillators to ensure this by the use of gel pads (Figure 3.6) or electrode cream and exerting firm pressure to the handles of the electrodes. One electrode is placed below the right clavicle in the midclavicular line, the other on the lower left chest

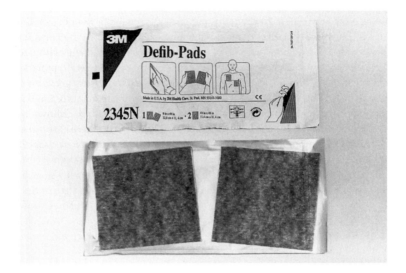

Figure 3.6 Defibrillation gel pads

outside the line of the cardiac apex taking care to avoid breast tissue in female subjects. If the conventional position is unsuccessful, other positions like the apex–posterior position may be considered. The polarity of the electrodes seems unimportant with external defibrillation. Care should be taken if the subject has had a pacemaker (or implanted defibrillator) placed in the area below the clavicle. The defibrillator electrodes should be placed at least 12.5 cm from the generator to minimize the risk of damage to the generator itself, or (by current travelling down the pacing wire and producing a burn at the point of contact with the endocardium) the subsequent loss of electrical capture.

Safety

The safety of those involved in the resuscitation attempt is a prime consideration. Before giving a shock the operator must shout 'stand clear' and ensure that nobody helping the resuscitation procedure has any contact with the patient before delivering the shock. Automated defibrillators give a verbal command to stand clear which must be obeyed. There are traps for the unwary: electrode gel, liquids or wet clothing must be avoided and special care is necessary when the patient is lying on a metallic or wet surface. Intravenous infusion equipment must not be held by helpers. The operator must also avoid all contact with the patient and the defibrillator electrodes. Care is also required to avoid excess electrode gel spreading across the precordium during chest compressions or electrical arcing between the electrodes may occur. Similarly, if gel is allowed to spread to the operator's hands arcing from the electrodes may occur. The use of special gel impregnated defibrillator pads greatly reduces this risk, and their use has much to commend it. With AEDs the adhesive electrodes feature integral gel pads and the risk does not arise. Finally transdermal drug administration patches should be removed to prevent electrical arcing due to a voltage breakdown occurring between an electrode and the patch.

Non-VF/VT rhythms

If VF/VT can definitely be excluded, defibrillation is not indicated and the right-hand side of the algorithm should be followed. These patients will either have asystole or electromechanical dissociation (EMD) (Figure 3.7). The prognosis is much less favourable than for patients in ventricular fibrillation, but the chances of success must not be discounted. Because ventricular fibrillation is so readily treatable it is vital that great care is taken before diagnosing asystole. With a manual defibrillator the position of the electrodes, the integrity of electrical connections and the gain of the monitor must all be checked. All contact with the patient must cease briefly to reduce the possibility of interference. An alternative position for the defibrillator electrodes should be employed or an alternative ECG lead should be monitored whenever possible. If there is any doubt that the rhythm might be ventricular fibrillation of low amplitude rather than asystole, then initial treatment should be as for ventricular fibrillation with attempts at defibrillation.

An automated defibrillator may not recognize fine ventricular fibrillation when the amplitude of the waveform is below the sensitivity of the instrument. Under these circumstances the machine will determine that no shock is indicated and time will be wasted. It is necessary to convert the defibrillator to a manual mode of operation before defibrillation can be carried out.

Although the prognosis of patients with EMD or asystole is much less favourable than in cases of ventricular fibrillation, the possibility of success should not be disregarded. This is particularly important when asystole is

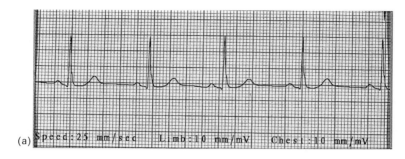

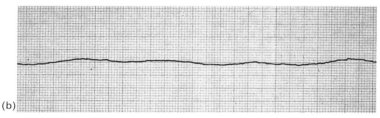

Figure 3.7 (a) Electromechanical dissociation and (b) asystole

the primary rhythm causing the arrest rather than the terminal rhythm following the degeneration of other rhythms. In some patients there are potentially reversible causes or aggravating factors in the causation of asystole or EMD and a search for and correction of these factors may result in success. A list of causes is included in the box at the foot of the algorithm and conveniently remembered as the '4Hs and the 4Ts'. During the assessment and possible treatment of these conditions 3 minutes of CPR should be given, during which the airway must be secured and ventilation and oxygenation are provided while attempts are made at gaining intravenous access. As with the management of ventricular fibrillation, adrenaline is given approximately every 3 minutes to increase the efficiency of basic life support.

Atropine is the only recommended drug treatment in the presence of asystole, and has been included in resuscitation guidelines for many years. Atropine has a well-established role in the treatment of bradycardia and heart block, but evidence for its use in asystole is less well founded. Increased vagal tone might contribute to the development of asystole or its unresponsiveness to treatment and atropine should be given once only during the first cycle of the loop in a dose sufficient to block vagal tone completely; 3 mg intravenously is the recommended dose. Adverse effects are unlikely in this situation, and there are anecdotal accounts as well as small clinical studies reporting success with its use in this now desperate situation.

After the first 3-minute cycle of CPR the patient's electrical rhythm is reassessed. If the rhythm has changed to one compatible with a cardiac output, the presence of a cardiac output should be assessed with a pulse check. If the rhythm has changed to ventricular fibrillation then the left-hand side of the algorithm is followed, otherwise loops of the right-hand side of the algorithm are followed for as long as it is considered appropriate to continue the resuscitation attempt. Resuscitation should usually continue for at least 20–30 minutes from the time of collapse unless there are overwhelming reasons to believe that continuing is futile. Resuscitation should not usually be abandoned while the rhythm is recognizably ventricular fibrillation or tachycardia.

Drug administration

Intravenous

The intravenous route is the most effective method of administering drugs during resuscitation attempts, but securing IV access may not be straightforward outside hospital. Paramedics in the UK carry the necessary equipment and practise the skill regularly, which is an additional advantage of involving the ambulance service at an early stage in the treatment of patients who may require resuscitation. Without help, basic life support will be interrupted for an unacceptable period while the necessary equipment is assembled and venous cannulation is attempted.

The antecubital fossa provides the best route of access to the venous circulation in most patients; only rarely will it be possible to undertake central venous catheterization outside hospital and the potential complication rate outweighs the (largely theoretical) advantages of central venous access in this situation.

Endobronchial

The endobronchial route offers an alternative method of administering drugs when a tracheal tube is in place. This is often the case when paramedics start resuscitation and perform tracheal intubation to gain control of the airway at an early stage. Adrenaline, atropine and lignocaine may all be given by this route; the dose is two to three times the intravenous route diluted in at least 10 ml of saline. The dose should preferably be given through a cannula that reaches to the distal end of the tracheal tube and five ventilations should be given to increase dispersion into the bronchial tree. This route is inferior to the venous route because absorption is unpredictable when the circulation is maintained purely by basic life support, particularly in the presence of pulmonary oedema. Nevertheless, it may be the only route available for drug administration outside hospital, and familiarity with the technique is useful.

Other routes

Intracardiac injection into the right ventricle approached from either the subxiphoid route or from between the fourth and fifth left intercostal cartilages is rarely carried out. The route is unreliable and post-mortem studies have shown that often the injection is not given into the heart at all. Damage to the ventricular myocardium and coronary arteries may occur, and pneumothorax and haemopericardium are additional complications. It is a last resort when no other route is possible.

The intraosseous route is considered in the chapter on paediatric resuscitation, as it is most commonly used in children.

Specific drug treatments

There is no overwhelming evidence that the use of drugs improves survival in humans who sustain a cardiac arrest outside hospital. Drugs have been used empirically because of known pharmacological effects that have been perceived to be potentially advantageous in cardiac arrest or because of evidence derived from animal experiments. Clinical trials in these circumstances are very difficult to conduct, and the evidence base for the use of drugs in clinical practice remains imperfect in many circumstances. The most important drugs are considered here.

Adrenaline and vasopressor drugs

Vasoconstrictor drugs are used during cardiopulmonary resuscitation to produce peripheral vasoconstriction. The increase in systemic vascular resistance raises the pressure in the aorta and thereby increases coronary profusion pressure. Differential shunting of blood also occurs to the cerebral circulation. The net result is an increase in perfusion within the coronary and cerebral circulations at the expense of decreased peripheral blood flow. There is considerable evidence from animal work that these effects are beneficial and lead to increased rates of resuscitation. Evidence that they increase rates of resuscitation in human cardiac arrest is less convincing and there is no strong evidence from placebo-controlled trials on which to base recommendations for dosage and frequency of administration.

The basic purpose of vasopressor drugs is to increase the efficiency of basic life support. Adrenaline is the drug recommended regardless of the mechanism of cardiac arrest. Adrenaline stimulates alpha one, alpha two, beta one and beta two adrenoceptors, but it is the effect on alpha receptors that is most important in this context. Beta stimulation may be detrimental as beta one receptor stimulation will lead to an increase in heart rate and force of contraction, which increases myocardial oxygen requirements. Beta two stimulation increases glycogenolysis which increases oxygen requirements and also produces hypokalaemia which may increase the chance of arrhythmias. To avoid the potentially detrimental effects of beta receptor stimulation selective alpha agonists have been investigated but have not been found to be effective in most trials.

The smooth muscle of the peripheral resistance vessels contains both alpha one and alpha two receptors which produce vasoconstriction in response to adrenaline. During hypoxia alpha two receptors are thought to contribute more towards vasomotor tone and this may explain the ineffectiveness of pure alpha one agonists. Adrenaline and noradrenaline, which have similar actions on alpha receptors, have been shown to enhance coronary perfusion pressure during cardiac arrest. The alpha two effects seem to become increasingly important as the duration of the arrest increases and some of the beta agonist activity may have beneficial effects in part by counteracting alpha-two-mediated coronary vasoconstriction. Several clinical trials have compared different vasoconstrictor agents but none has been shown to be more effective than adrenaline, which retains its place in modern resuscitation guidelines.

Experimental work in animals has suggested that higher doses of adrenaline may be more effective, but clinical trials in humans have not confirmed this. In one trial, a dose of 5 mg of adrenaline in patients with asystolic or electromechanical disassociation was associated with a higher initial success rate when compared with the standard dose of 1 mg but, unfortunately, the hospital discharge rate was not improved. Detrimental effects of high catecholamine levels include arrhythmias, sustained myocardial contraction and necrosis, increased myocardial oxygen demands, coronary vasoconstriction and hypertension after successful resuscitation.

Atropine

Atropine antagonizes acetylcholine (the parasympathetic neurotransmitter) at muscarinic receptors. The most important in the present context are those in the vagus nerve. By reducing vagal tone in the heart sinus node automaticity is increased and atrioventricular conduction through the AV node is augmented. Although the use of atropine in the treatment of bradyarrhythmias due to increased parasympathetic tone is well founded in other situations – for example the increased parasympathetic tone that may accompany myocardial infarction – it has never conclusively been shown to be of benefit in asystolic cardiac arrest. The anecdotal accounts of success after its administration and limited trial evidence support its inclusion in the guidelines and it should be given once only, in a dose of 3 mg which is adequate to block vagal tone completely.

Antiarrhythmic drugs

In the circumstances under discussion these are used to terminate malignant arrhythmias, to facilitate electrical defibrillation and to prevent recurrence of ventricular fibrillation or tachycardia. Several agents have been investigated, lignocaine the most extensively. Several trials have shown that lignocaine is effective in preventing the occurrence of ventricular defibrillation after acute infarction, but these were conducted in a setting where defibrillation was readily available and overall mortality was not improved by the use of lignocaine. Its effectiveness in preventing ventricular fibrillation has been extrapolated to suggest that it may be effective in treating ventricular fibrillation, particularly in conjunction with electrical defibrillation. Studies on animals, however, have consistently shown that the energy levels required for defibrillation is increased when lignocaine is given and, in one trial in humans, there was a threefold greater occurrence of asystole after defibrillation when lignocaine had been administered.

Other drugs including bretylium and amiodarone have been advocated and both are currently the subjects of clinical trials. At present there are inadequate data to advocate their use for any of the roles suggested in the treatment of ventricular fibrillation.

Conclusions

Adrenaline should be present in all emergency bags because of its undoubted role in the treatment of anaphylaxis and so it should be available for use during resuscitation attempts in the community. There is a sound theoretical basis for its use supported by experimental work performed in animals. It retains its place in current guidelines and it is hoped that further research will define its role more precisely and establish optimal doses and treatment regimens.

Atropine should also be carried in the emergency bag to treat symptomatic bradycardia, particularly the haemodynamic effects of vagally-induced bradycardia following acute myocardial infarctions. For this purpose doses lower than the 3 mg recommended for asystolic cardiac arrest are required – five of the convential $600\,\mu g$ ampoules would be necessary.

There is no strong scientific basis for the use of antiarrhythmic agents in the routine management of cardiac arrest outside hospital. Lignocaine is the drug likely to be available but will only very infrequently be used in the treatment of ventricular fibrillation. Its use in the treatment of ventricular tachycardia in the presence of a cardiac output is a separate issue beyond the scope of this chapter.

Alkalizing agents, traditionally sodium bicarbonate, have been used in resuscitation attempts in an attempt to reverse the metabolic and respiratory acidosis that occurs. Much of the evidence for the use of alkalizing agents and buffers has been derived from animal work and studies in humans have tended to concentrate on patients with prolonged cardiac arrest where resuscitation was unlikely to have been successful. It has also proved difficult to isolate the effect of the alkalizing agent from the adrenaline given concurrently – the effect of the latter being enhanced by correction of the pH. There are many potentially disadvantageous effects likely to follow the administration of sodium bicarbonate including worsening of intracellular acidosis and the adverse consequences of the hyperosmolar sodium load.

Current guidelines recommend the use of alkalizing agents under controlled conditions with the benefit of blood gas analysis. The primary health care team need concern themselves no further!

References and further reading

Bossaert L, Callanan V, Cummins RO (1997) Early defibrillation; an advisory statement by the Advanced Life Support Working Group of the International Liaison Committee on resuscitation. *Resuscitation,* **34**:113–14.

Colquhoun MC, Camm AJ (1999) Asystole and electromechanical dissociation. In *ABC of Resuscitation* 4th edn. (Colquhoun MC, Handley AJ, Evans T, eds) pp 5–10. BMJ Books, London.

Colquhoun MC (1999) Drugs and their delivery. In *ABC of Resuscitation* 4th edn. (Colquhoun MC, Handley AJ, Evans T, eds) pp 5–10. BMJ Books, London.

Colquhoun MC, Chamberlain D A (1999) Ventricular fibrillation. In *ABC of Resuscitation* 4th edn. (Colquhoun MC, Handley AJ, Evans T, eds) pp 5–10. BMJ Books, London.

European Resuscitation Council (1992) Guidelines for advanced life support. A statement by the Advanced Life Support Working Party of the European Resuscitation Council. *Resuscitation,* **24**:111–21.

European Resuscitation Council (1998) The 1998 European Resuscitation Council guidelines for adult advanced life support, pp 36–47. *European Resuscitation Council Guidelines for Resuscitation* (Bossaert L, ed.). Elsevier, Oxford.

Kloeck W, Cummins R, Chamberlain D *et al.* (1997) The Universal ALS; an advisory statement by the Advanced Life Support Working Group of the International Liaison Committee on resuscitation. *Resuscitation,* **34**:109–11.

Nolan J (1998) The 1998 European Resuscitation Council guidelines for adult advanced life support. *BMJ,* **316**:1863–9.

Vincent R (1997) Drugs in modern resuscitation. *British Journal of Anesthesia,* **79**:188–97.

Chapter 4

Management of the airway and ventilation

The maintenance of a patent airway and the provision of ventilation in a patient who is unable to do this for himself (or herself), for whatever reason, are important life-saving skills that should be possessed by any GP.

The main objectives of airway management before hospital admission are to provide the patient with a patent airway, provide oxygenation to prevent or reverse hypoxia and to protect the lungs from the risk of aspiration. In this chapter we discuss some of the principles involved with airway management, particularly in relation to practice outside hospital, and consider the methods available. As in any other branch of emergency medical care, a familiarity with techniques and confidence in their application are the important issues.

Airway obstruction

The airway will become obstructed when the base of the tongue falls backwards to cover the larynx. This most commonly happens when the unconscious patient is lying supine, but it may also occur with patients lying prone or in the lateral position. Abnormal muscular activity within the tongue and upper airway results in a failure to maintain adequate airway patency when the head is in a neutral or flexed position. Other causes of airway obstruction include foreign bodies, fluids (for example vomit, secretions and blood) or oedema in the upper airway.

Whatever the cause of the obstruction, it is most important that it is identified and treated effectively. The presence of airway obstruction is usually recognized by the absence of ventilation in a patient who is making respiratory efforts, or by a failure to inflate the chest of a patient who is unconscious and not breathing.

It is important to adopt a systematic approach to the assessment of patients with an obstructed airway. With partial airway obstruction the breathing is usually noisy. Stridor is the term used to describe the inspiratory noise heard in patients with obstruction of the upper airways (the airways lying above the thoracic inlet, for practical purposes the oropharynx, pharynx and larynx). An expiratory wheeze suggests obstruction of the more distal airways. The causes and significance of the two are quite distinct and require different approaches to treatment. Gurgling is heard when fluid is present in large airways and will indicate the need for suction. Snoring occurs when the pharynx is partially occluded, usually by the tongue or soft palate.

Complete airway obstruction may be accompanied by vigorous inspiratory efforts with the accessory muscles of respiration in the neck and shoulders used to assist expansion of the thorax. As the patient attempts to breathe in, the chest wall rises but the abdomen is drawn inwards — a reversal of the normal pattern whereby the abdomen moves outwards during inspiration, pushed down by the diaphragm as the lungs expand. Auscultation will reveal the absence of breath sounds.

Manoeuvres to open and clear the airway

Head tilt/chin lift

This procedure (Figure 4.1) (which is described in the chapter on Basic Life Support) is a core skill that should be possessed by all health care workers who have patient contact. By exerting traction on the anterior tissues of the neck the tongue is displaced forward away from the posterior pharyngeal wall. It is an effective method of opening the airway in an unconscious patient and airway patency can be achieved by this simple technique in around 90% of cases.

Jaw thrust

The jaw thrust is an alternative procedure for displacing the mandible anteriorly to relieve obstruction caused by the tongue. It is the best technique in patients in whom cervical spine injury is suspected as it is not necessary to tilt the head backwards with the inherent danger of cord damage occurring from movement of the cervical spine. Ideally, the jaw thrust technique should be combined with manual in-line stabilization of the head and neck performed by an assistant who maintains the head in the neutral position. To perform the jaw thrust, kneel at the head of the

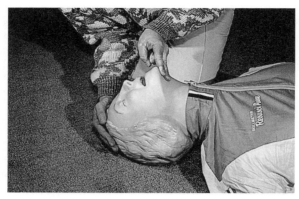

Figure 4.1 Head tilt, chin lift

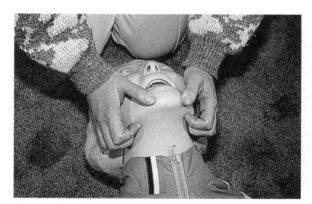

Figure 4.2 Jaw thrust

casualty and identify the ankle of the jaw (mandible). Place the index and other fingers behind the angle and apply steady upwards and forwards pressure to lift the jaw and open the airway. Use the thumbs to open the mouth by displacing the chin downwards (Figure 4.2).

Whichever technique is used, check for success by looking, listening and feeling for air movement. If a clear airway cannot be maintained by these techniques other causes of airway obstruction must be considered. A finger sweep should be performed to remove a solid foreign body but, in most cases, more advanced techniques requiring special equipment will be required.

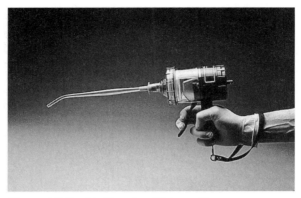

Figure 4.3 Hand-held suction (Vitalograph)

Adjuncts to basic airway techniques

Suction

When vomit or secretions are present in the upper airways, suction will usually be required. A number of portable suction devises are available and a rigid Yankauer sucker will enable the clearance of large volumes of fluid from the mouth and pharynx (Figure 4.3). A flexible catheter can be used to perform suction in the more distal airways. Ventilation may be compromised if suction is unduly prolonged and it should not usually need to be performed for longer than about 10 seconds.

A number of portable suction units are available; cost, ease of transport and power source will usually determine which model is chosen. For use by general practitioners outside hospital, the authors favour mechanical suction devices that do not require batteries or a source of mains electricity. Inexpensive, robust and reliable models are available that are suited for prolonged periods of storage between use (Figure 4.4).

Oropharyngeal and nasopharyngeal airways

Oropharyngeal and nasopharyngeal airways are designed to overcome airway obstruction caused by tongue displacement (Figure 4.5). Both provide a conduit to permit the passage of air between the tongue and posterior pharyngeal wall. Both also require the position of the head and neck to be maintained so that the alignment of the airway is ensured. In many cases head tilt or jaw thrust may also be required.

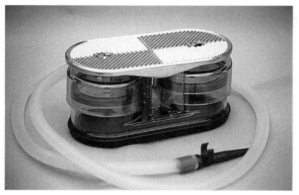

Figure 4.4 Foot pump (Medtronic)

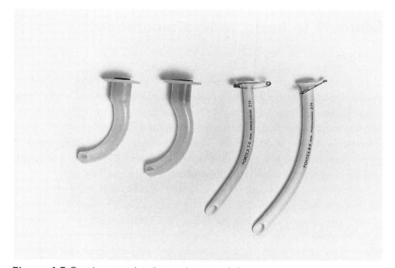

Figure 4.5 Oropharyngeal and nasopharyngeal airways

Oropharyngeal (Guedal) airway

The oropharyngeal or Guedel airway is a curved plastic tube flattened in the anterior-posterior dimension to provide a neat fit between the tongue and palate. It is reinforced at the oral end with a flange that fits against the patient's lips.

This airway can only be used in a patient who is unconscious and in whom the upper airway reflexes are absent, otherwise vomiting or laryngeal spasm may be induced.

An appropriately sized airway holds the tongue in the normal anatomical position and follows its natural curvature. The correct size is estimated by selecting an airway whose length corresponds to the distance between the angle of the jaw and the corner of the mouth. A considerable range of sizes is available for newborn, paediatric and adult subjects. The most commonly used sizes in adults are 2, 3 and 4, designed for small, medium and large subjects respectively.

These devices are relatively cheap and pre-packed sterile models are available.

Procedure for insertion

The casualty's mouth should be opened; ensure there are no foreign bodies or other material likely to be pushed more distally into the airway.

The airway is inserted into the mouth in the inverted position and, as it passes over the soft palate, it is rotated through 180 degrees to bring the distal end into position in the oropharynx at the back of the tongue. The patient must be unconscious to employ this technique and, if any reflexes are seen, the procedure should be abandoned.

Correct placement is confirmed by the establishment of a patent airway confirmed by the usual look, listen and feel technique while maintaining the position of the head and neck. The position of the airway should be checked periodically to ensure that it does not become displaced.

Nasopharyngeal airway

The nasopharayngeal airway is a tube made of soft malleable plastic with a bevel at one end and a flange at the other. It is usually better tolerated than the Guedel airway in patients who are less deeply unconscious, and has particular value in patients where oral access is not possible because of injury or trismus.

Determining the correct size

It is important to choose an airway of the correct size because if it is too small it will be ineffective, while if it is too long it may cause laryngospasm or vomiting. Tubes of various diameters are available, the length increasing

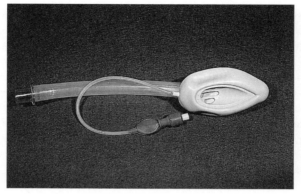

Figure 4.6 Laryngeal mask airway

with the diameter. A 6–8 mm tube will be suitable for most adults and, as a rough guide, the diameter should be the same as the thickness of the casualty's little finger.

Procedure for insertion

Having ensured that the right nostril is patent, the lubricated tube is inserted with the bevelled end first. It is passed downwards along the floor of the nasal cavity and by using a slight twisting action is manipulated into the posterior pharynx. It is customary to insert a safety pin through the tube near the flange to prevent the tube being inhaled and once in place a tape may be used to secure it. When in position the patency of the airway must be ensured using the usual look, listen and feel approach. It is also important to maintain correct alignment of the head and airway.

The nasopharyngeal airway is inexpensive and relatively straightforward to use and therefore quite appropriate for inclusion in the practice emergency kit. Although likely to be used only very infrequently, it may be life saving.

Laryngeal mask airway

The laryngeal mask airway (LMA) (Figure 4.6) was invented by an English anaesthetist Archie Brain and introduced in the early 1980s. It has revolutionized anaesthetic practice in this country and is increasingly used in resuscitation attempts in hospital. It provides many of the advantages of tracheal intubation but is an easier technique to perform requiring less training and less equipment. Clinical studies have shown that it may be used effectively by nurses and others likely to be present in the early stages of a resuscitation attempt on a hospital ward. Its use is spreading outside the hospital environment and increasingly, paramedics are being trained in its operation. The laryngeal mask airway is certainly a practical alternative to the tracheal tube for most situations likely to be encountered by the primary health care team.

Although more expensive than the tracheal tube, fewer sizes are required and its use is not dependent on the laryngoscope (with the attendant risks of bulb or battery failure after the periods of storage between the use that is likely in primary care). It may also be re-sterilized and used repeatedly.

The laryngeal mask airway consists of a curved tube with an inflatable cuff at one end. When inflated, the cuff seals round the laryngeal opening enabling ventilation to be performed while at the same time offering protection against aspiration.

The laryngeal mask is a safe and reliable method of providing ventilation and is more efficient than a bag/valve/mask device. Although it does not provide the same degree of airway protection as tracheal intubation, it can be inserted easily with a high success rate after comparatively little training. Pulmonary aspiration is uncommon with the laryngeal mask and, provided high inflation pressures are avoided, gastric inflation is minimal. The device can usually be inserted with relatively little movement of the head and neck which offers an advantage when cervical spine injury is suspected.

The laryngeal mask used in anaesthetic practice may be sterilized and used repeatedly. Recently a pre-packed sterile disposable version has been introduced designed for single use. This may offer some advantages for the pre-hospital practitioner.

There has not yet been much published experience of the use of the LMA outside hospital, but most reports have been favourable. The technique of insertion is normally easy to acquire and its use is usually straightforward in patients with impaired consciousness.

Technique for insertion

Select an appropriately sized LMA (usually size 4 or 5 for adults). Ensure the cuff is deflated and adequately lubricated. The operator should kneel at the head of the patient placed in a supine position with the head and neck in alignment. Ideally the neck should be slightly flexed and the head extended (the sniffing the morning air position), but neck movements must be avoided if cervical spine injury is a possibility. The tube is introduced into the mouth and advanced with the open surface uppermost to the posterior pharyngeal area. The mask is then rotated and advanced backwards and downwards until resistance is felt as the tip locates in the hypopharynx. The cuff is then inflated with the specified amount of air and the tube will lift slightly out of the mouth (1–2 cm). Correct positioning can be confirmed by listening for breath sounds during inflation and observing chest movement. The proximal end of the tube incorporates a standard fitting enabling connection to the equipment used to ventilate the patient, usually a bag/valve/mask device. Once in position it is usual to place something alongside the tube (e.g. a Guedal airway) to prevent the patient biting on the tube. It can be secured in position with a bandage.

Complications may occur if the patient is not deeply unconscious because pharyngeal stimulation may induce vomiting or laryngospasm, but this is not an issue in the context of cardiopulmonary arrest. Airway obstruction may result, particularly if the epiglottis is pushed downwards to cover the laryngeal inlet. So, if chest inflation is unsuccessful (as it will be in this situation), the cuff must be deflated and the tube withdrawn before a further attempt at insertion is made.

The Combitube

The combitube is a double lumen airway introduced blindly over the tongue and advanced towards the larynx. The tube usually enters the oesophagus and the patient is ventilated through the oesophageal channel by openings in the tube a few centimetres proximal to the tip (which is sealed). A cuff proximal to the blind end acts as further protection against gastric inflation. A further cuff inflated in the hypopharynx helps ensure air passes into the lungs.

If the tube enters the trachea, ventilation is provided directly through the tracheal channel which has an open end. The device has achieved some popularity in the USA and Europe and has been successfully employed by paramedics. It has not gained widespread popularity in the UK, but its use may become more widespread in the future and it is mentioned for this reason.

Tracheal intubation

Tracheal intubation is still considered the best method of protecting the airway and providing ventilation. The inflated cuff at the distal end of the tube prevents the possibility of aspiration of gastric contents and enables ventilation to be achieved without leaks even when increased inflation pressures are required, for example in severe acute asthma or pulmonary oedema. Catheters may be passed through the tube to perform suction of the distal airways or to administer drugs.

Tracheal intubation requires considerable training and experience and skills are likely to deteriorate unless the procedure is performed on a regular basis. Deterioration in the patient's condition may occur if ventilation is interrupted for a prolonged period while the tube is inserted and it is important that this is avoided by pre-oxygenating the patient before attempting insertion, and not persisting for undue periods if insertion proves difficult. Further oxygenation should be provided in this scenario before trying again. Paramedics in the UK are taught endotracheal intubation and undergo regular re-training and practice in hospitals to maintain skill levels. This would not usually be possible for members of the primary health care team unless anaesthetic training has been undertaken and experience is continued through a hospital attachment; for most GPs therefore, it will not be appropriate to perform tracheal intubation. Most patients may be ventilated initially by simpler techniques and the need for tracheal intubation can be considered in conjunction with the ambulance service. For this reason, the techniques of tracheal intubation will not be considered in detail in this book and readers who wish to learn more about the technique should consult textbooks on anaesthesia.

There are many other problems with the practice of endotracheal intubation, particularly outside hospital. The use of the laryngoscope and the insertion of the tube will increase the risk of regurgitation (and consequently aspiration) in all patients. In patients with head injury, laryngoscopy may increase intracranial pressure. The inherent difficulties of performing endotracheal intubation outside hospital make the possibility of oesophageal intubation, which is a disaster, increasingly likely. Sedative or paralysing drugs are often required to permit successful intubation in hospital practice and the use of these agents in the pre-hospital environment is fraught with difficulties. In the context of trauma, there is evidence that if endotracheal intubation is possible without the use of sedative or paralysing drugs the prognosis is very poor indeed.

In patients with cardiac arrest, the time taken to perform intubation (when chest compression will be interrupted) is a significant factor and, in the majority of patients, adequate ventilation may be provided by much simpler techniques.

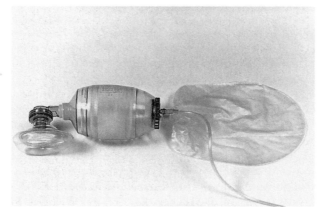

Figure 4.7 Self-inflating bag device (disposable models available for under £20)

Ventilation

Artificial ventilation must be commenced as soon as possible in any patient in whom spontaneous breathing is inadequate or absent. Expired air ventilation either by mouth-to-mouth ventilation or by using a pocket mask is an effective holding procedure, but the concentration of inspired oxygen is only around 16% and it is important to increase this as soon as practicable. This may be possible with the pocket mask with models that feature a side port which allows the connection of oxygen. The subject of expired air ventilation is considered in the chapter on basic life support and in this section we are primarily concerned with the use of special equipment to assist the ventilation of a casualty.

Self-inflating bag

This is the device most commonly used to ventilate patients. It can be connected to a pocket mask, the anaesthetist's facemask, the laryngeal mask airway or a tracheal tube through a universal fitting.

In principle the self-inflating bag is a simple device (Figure 4.7). When the bag is squeezed its contents are delivered to the patient and the return of exhaled gas is prevented by a one-way valve. The bag refills automatically via an inlet usually situated at the opposite end to the exit point.

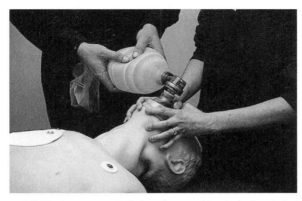

Figure 4.8 The two-person technique for use of bag/valve/mask device

Although the self-inflating bag appears straightforward it requires considerable skill to use it effectively. When used with a facemask for example, it is difficult to achieve an adequate seal on the patient's face while simultaneously maintaining the airway with one hand, and squeezing the bag with the other. The equipment is often best used as a two-operator technique with one operator applying the facemask and maintaining the airway while the other squeezes the bag (Figure 4.8). Over-inflation will result in gastric distension and inadequate squeezing will result in hypoventilation. Most of these problems can be reduced by connecting the bag to an LMA or tracheal tube to eliminate leaks and ensure that gas is only delivered to the lungs.

Oxygen may be connected directly to the bag to increase the concentration of inspired oxygen from that of room air (21%) to around 50%. Much higher concentrations of inspired oxygen may be achieved by the use of a reservoir bag connected to the inlet. This is filled from the oxygen supply and concentrations of inspired oxygen of 90% may be achieved.

Mechanical ventilators

A number of small portable automatic ventilators are available and are widely carried by the ambulance service. The majority are gas powered with oxygen from a cylinder being used both to supply the patient and to power the ventilator. The volume of gas delivered during inspiration is controlled by the inspiratory time. The devices are pressure limited to protect the lungs from barotrauma but very high airway pressures may develop if chest compression coincides with inspiration. The risk of such barotrauma is reduced by a pressure limitation device, but inadequate ventilation may then result. In general their use cannot be recommended for the occasional user and they are not really suitable for use by the primary care team unless considerable training has been undertaken.

Surgical airway

It may prove impossible to ventilate the patient with a bag/valve/mask or to pass an LMA or tracheal tube. This may occur with facial trauma (not a common problem in primary care); mechanical obstruction of the larynx by inhaled foreign bodies or the epiglottis are other possible causes. Needle cricothyroidotomy is the most appropriate technique outside hospital in this situation. It has definite advantages over tracheostomy which requires considerable surgical skill and special equipment and is time consuming. To perform needle cricothyroidotomy, the patient is placed supine with the head slightly extended. The cricothyroid membrane between the thyroid and cricoid cartilage is identified by palpation and punctured with a large bore cannula. The aspiration of air confirms the correct position in the trachea. The cannula is then advanced further and the needle is removed. The cannula is ideally attached to a high pressure oxygen supply via a Y connector, oxygenation being performed by occluding the open limb of the Y. It is also possible to feed a guide wire down the cannula. Once placed in the trachea the cannula is removed and a dilator is fed over the guide wire and passed distally through the skin into the airway. Once the track has been created a tubular airway placed on the dilator may be advanced into the airway. When in position the dilator and guide wire are removed to leave the cricothyrotomy tube in place enabling the patient to be ventilated with oxygen. The diameter of this airway is considerably larger than an intravenous cannula and ventilation may be carried out more easily and effectively.

The procedure may be carried out quickly and is relatively straight-forward to perform. This technique, as well as needle cricothyrotomy, are only holding procedures until a definitive airway can be established in hospital; they will be used very infrequently in primary care but may, nevertheless, be life saving.

Cricoid pressure

Cricoid pressure was first described by Sellick in 1961. He advocated its use during the induction of anaesthesia to reduce the incidence of aspiration of gastric contents. More recently it has been recommended during resuscitation attempts, particularly in late pregnancy, until the airway can be protected by other means. The high incidence of pulmonary aspiration during cardiac arrests emphasizes the need for all practitioners to be aware of the value of cricoid pressure during resuscitation and be competent and safe at administering it.

Mode of action

Performed correctly, cricoid pressure will occlude the lumen of the oesophagus; this will have a two-fold effect preventing:

- regurgitation and aspiration of gastric contents
- inflation of the stomach during ventilation, particularly when a bag/valve/mask is used.

Technique

1. Locate the cricoid cartilage – the first complete ring of cartilage below the thyroid cartilage (Adam's apple).
2. Place the index finger and thumb on either side of the cricoid cartilage.
3. Apply backward pressure to obstruct the lumen of the oesophagus lying posteriorly. (Counterpressure may also be applied at the back of the neck, but this is *not* recommended when cervical spine injury is suspected).
4. Pressure should only be released when the airway is protected, for example by a cuffed tracheal tube (or if the casualty actively vomits).

Cautions

- Cricoid pressure should not be applied during active vomiting because there is a risk of damage to the oesophagus
- The anatomy of the airway can be distorted if too much pressure is applied and this will hinder tracheal intubation.

References and further references

European Resuscitation Council (1998) *The 1998 ERC guidelines for the management of the airway and ventilation during resuscitation in European Resuscitation Council Guidelines for Resuscitation* (Bossaert L, ed.) Elsevier, Oxford.

Simons R (1999) The airway at risk. In *ABC of Resuscitation,* 4th edn (Colquhoun MC, Handley AJ, Evans T, eds), p. 19–24. BMJ Books, London.

Chapter 5

Resuscitation in special circumstances

There are a number of specific situations where resuscitation is carried out but the procedures are adapted to suit the circumstances and requirements of the patient. Cardiopulmonary arrest caused by poisoning, hypothermia and near drowning are examples, and although it is rare for a member of the practice team to attempt resuscitation under these circumstances, a doctor or nurse present at such an emergency will be expected to know what to do, furthermore their actions may prove lifesaving. The purpose of this chapter is to provide guidance about what to do in these situations and our recommendations are based on the guidelines published by the authoritative bodies in the field.

Near drowning

The term 'near drowning' is used to describe successful resuscitation after asphyxiation by fluid. The main effect of submersion is the cessation of effective respiration with cardiac arrest occurring as a secondary event; hypothermia is a frequent accompaniment and may be advantageous as it helps preserve neurological function. The circulation may continue for some time after immersion, and successful resuscitation after prolonged periods of immersion has been reported, particularly in children apparently drowned in cold water. Survival has been reported after submersion for periods as long as 1 hour and prolonged resuscitation attempts are justified in these circumstances.

The initial treatment is the same regardless of whether salt water or fresh water is involved. No modifications of basic life support techniques are required, but it is important to be aware of the possibility of cervical spine injury associated with diving accidents, particularly in shallow water. It is almost impossible to perform basic life support while the patient is in the water, although some rescue breaths may be attempted. The rescuer should not attempt to drain water from the lungs, but foreign bodies present in the airway should be removed. The casualty should be placed in a horizontal position to aid the drainage of water and to reduce the risks of the postural hypotension that commonly follow the removal of the patient who has been immersed in water for a prolonged period. This occurs because the hydrostatic pressure exerted by the water causes the redistribution of fluid within body compartments, and circulatory collapse may result when the victim is removed from the water and this pressure is removed.

Ventilation with 100% oxygen should be started as soon as possible and tracheal intubation offers many advantages if the expertise and equipment is available. Pulmonary aspiration following vomiting or regurgitation is common in this situation and tracheal intubation protects the airway and enables more efficient ventilation. High inflation pressures may be required – an additional advantage of tracheal intubation.

Basic life support should be carried out according to standard guidelines, but it is important to be aware that hypothermia frequently accompanies immersion injury, and particular care is necessary before deciding that the pulse is absent; the presence of bradycardia contributes to this difficulty. The special considerations that apply to the management of cardiac arrhythmias in the presence of hypothermia are considered in a later section.

Effective resuscitation at the scene of the incident is paramount in determining the likelihood of success with the long-term survival of a neurologically intact patient. Few patients transferred to hospital with cardiopulmonary arrest survive, but there is currently increased interest in the treatment of profoundly hypothermic patients in special units. Success following re-warming on cardiopulmonary bypass is being reported with increasing frequency.

After initial resuscitation there is a danger of the subsequent development of pulmonary oedema – a type of acute respiratory distress syndrome. All patients should therefore be admitted to hospital for a period of observation after resuscitation. If bronchospasm is present (which may indicate the presence of aspirated fluid or the presence of pulmonary oedema), nebulized bronchodilators (for example salbutamol) should be given. In practice this should be relatively easy as most ambulances now carry nebulizers with salbutamol, if indeed the doctor does not have this in his own emergency equipment.

Hypothermia

By common agreement hypothermia is said to be present when the core body temperature falls below 35°C. It may occur in a variety of situations — exposure to adverse weather conditions is one common cause and hypothermia often follows immersion incidents. Hypothermia may follow prolonged unconsciousness associated with alcohol or drug intoxication and may sometimes be seen in patients unconscious for other reasons, like stroke, trauma or injury. It should be suspected from the circumstances in which the patient is found and confirmed by measurement of the temperature. This in itself presents some problems, particularly outside hospital where the measurement of rectal temperature is often impractical; in addition it does not always truly reflect the core body temperature. Modern electronic devices that measure the temperature from the tympanic membrane in the ear are now increasingly available at an economical price and are used by some GPs routinely to measure temperature. They are convenient in use as they do not require sterilization and give accurate readings as low as 20°C very quickly. They are probably the best practical method of assessing the core temperature outside hospital currently available.

The technique of basic life support should allow for the fact that hypothermia produces bradycardia and a slow ventilatory rate. It therefore is important to allow adequate time to confirm the absence of breathing or a pulse. Further heat loss to the environment should be prevented; wet garments should be removed and the patient should be removed from the cold environment or adverse weather conditions if possible.

Oxygen should be administered and this preferably should be warmed and humidified — portable apparatus that permits this is available and may be carried by the ambulance service. Rough movements and excessive activity should be avoided as these may precipitate ventricular fibrillation.

Where the pulse and breathing are present, arrangements should be made to transport the patient to hospital and active external re-warming can be applied to the truncal areas. External re-warming should not be used if cardiopulmonary arrest has occurred and in this situation basic life support should be initiated using the standard techniques. The rates for ventilation and chest compressions are the same as in the normothermic patient but may be more difficult to carry out if hypothermia has produced stiffness of the chest wall. Once basic life support has been started it should not usually be stopped until the patient has been re-warmed.

As body temperature falls, sinus bradycardia is followed by atrial fibrillation and later ventricular fibrillation. Asystole is the final end point. The universal ALS algorithm should be followed, but it is important to remember that ventricular fibrillation is very much harder to convert to sinus rhythm in the presence of hypothermia. If the core temperature is less than 30°C defibrillation may be impossible, and ERC guidelines recommend a maximum of three shocks for VF/VT in patients with a core temperature of less than 30°C and if these are unsuccessful further shocks should only be adminstered when the core temperature has been increased. Obviously basic life support must be continued during this period – successful resuscitation has been reported after 70 minutes of cardiac arrest followed by 2 hours of basic life support before active re-warming was initiated on cardiopulmonary bypass. The metabolism of drugs administered to hypothermic patients occurs more slowly than normal and it is usually recommended that intravenous medications are given at longer than standard intervals.

Once the patient has been stabilized in the field, arrangements should be made for transfer to hospital, preferably to a unit with the experience and equipment required. Unlike most patients who experience cardiopulmonary arrest in the community, the hypothermic patient has much to gain from transfer to hospital after initial attempts at resuscitation at the scene have not succeeded. Active internal re-warming may be started in the field but requires specialized knowledge and equipment; it may be appropriate to start this when the journey is likely to be prolonged. This may occur for example, after rescue in a remote location, but the institution of such treatment must not delay the transport of the patient to hospital where more advanced re-warming techniques are available.

Poisoning and drug intoxication

Although poisoning is a frequent cause of medical admissions to hospital only around 1–2% of patients have been exposed to sufficient toxin to be at a serious risk. Nevertheless, poisoning, by drugs or other toxic substances, is the second most common cause of death in the 18–35 years age range. The challenge to those providing pre-hospital care is to identify those at significant risk of developing cardiopulmonary arrest and treat them effectively to prevent this. In other some supportive treatment, particularly of the airway and ventilation, while transferring the patient to hospital may prove life saving.

The assessment of the poisoned patients

The most common situation seen in general practice is in patients poisoned by agents that have been injected or ingested.

Basic life support follows standard guidelines but a risk to the rescuer arises if the patient is infected with hepatitis B, C or HIV and a careful examination should be made for signs of intravenous drug abuse. The basic principles of restoring ventilation and oxygenation and providing circulation through basic life support remain the first priority; obstruction of the upper airway is one of the most common causes of death in patients dying from poisoning outside hospital. Mouth-to-mouth ventilation should be avoided if toxins like cyanide, organophosphates or corrosive substances are a possibility; the patient should be ventilated with a facemask or bag/valve/mask. Oxygen should be given in high concentration in nearly all circumstances, but paraquat poisoning is an exception to this rule because pulmonary injury may be increased by high concentrations of inspired oxygen.

There is a high incidence of pulmonary aspiration after poisoning and there are many advantages to be gained from early tracheal intubation. Intubation is essential before performing gastric lavage or administering activated charcoal in patients with severely depressed levels of consciousness.

Identification of toxin

One key role of those providing treatment of poisoned patients outside hospital is to try to identify the toxins responsible and provide samples whenever possible. An accurate history is essential and must be communicated to those providing the subsequent care. Patients will often admit the number and type of tablets taken but this information must be treated with caution as studies have shown that these statements do not always correlate with the findings of later toxicological analysis. Any medication, empty bottles or blister packs should be noted and sent with the patient to hospital. It is useful to establish whether the patient has vomited as this may reduce the potential dose of toxin absorbed. If the patient is unconscious it is important to think of other possible causes or contributing factors particularly hypoglycaemia, head injury or intracranial haemorrhage.

Any patient who has been exposed to a significant dose of toxin should be referred to hospital for further evaluation regardless of their initial clinical state. All patients who have taken drugs with suicidal intent must also be referred for psychiatric evaluation. In most cases the responsibility for ongoing supervision and treatment of the patient will rest with the ambulance service. Cardiac monitoring en route to hospital should be provided for any patient who is unconscious and for all patients known to have taken drugs likely to produce cardiac arrhythmia, for example beta blockers, calcium channel blockers, tricyclic antidepressants, antihistamines, or antiarrhythmic agents. It is also recommended that patients with pre-existing heart disease or who have inhalation injury should be monitored

.

Preventing absorption

There are obvious advantages in preventing the absorption of ingested poisons. The method currently recommended is the use of activated charcoal provided that it can be administered within 1–2 hours after ingestion; later administration greatly reduces its ability to prevent the absorption of toxin. Activated charcoal absorbs toxins onto its large surface area and is most effective while the toxin is still in the stomach. In some countries activated charcoal is widely employed as first aid treatment for poisoning by ingested substances before hospital admission. This is not commonly performed in the UK but deserves to become more widespread practice as early administration has the potential to be of great benefit to seriously poisoned patients. Furthermore, it is a particularly effective treatment for some of the drugs most commonly taken in overdosage — paracetamol, tricyclic antidepressants and anticonvulsants. For administration the patient should be conscious and should not be vomiting or fitting as this increases the risk of aspiration. It is not effective (and therefore should not be used) with many low molecular weight compounds like iron, lithium, cyanide, methanol, ethanol and ethylene glycol.

Traditional methods of inducing vomiting to reduce the absorption of toxins have been abandoned. Although syrup of ipecac is effective in inducing vomiting, it has not been shown to alter mortality in formal studies. If the induced vomiting persists, the administration of charcoal will be delayed or rendered less effective. Mechanical methods of inducing vomiting, for example by stimulating the oropharynx, are unreliable and not without risk. The other traditional method of inducing vomiting by the use of salt-containing drinks is associated with a very real risk of hypernatraemia and fatalities (in both adults and children) have been described.

Antidotes

The most important specific antidote is naloxone used in the case of opiate intoxication. It is worth remembering that opiates may be ingested (or injected) in many forms and overdoses involving a mixture of drugs are relatively common.

An unconscious apnoeic woman who had taken an overdose of several different drugs including co-proxamol (which contains dextropropoxyphene) rapidly starting breathing soon after an injection of naloxone given by one of the authors (MCC).

The half-life of the naloxone is shorter than that of the opiate drugs that it antagonizes and repeated intravenous doses may be required. An alternative strategy is to give half the dose intravenously and the remaining half intramuscularly to prolong its effect. Nevertheless, the effect of the drug may wear off during the journey to hospital and further dosages may be required. There are other potential problems with its use – the patient may wake up in an agitated state and refuse further treatment or admission and, for this reason, some authorities do not recommend the use of naloxone outside hospital unless there is potentially life-threatening opiate poisoning with severe depression of respiration (less than 8 breaths per minute) or where consciousness is severely impaired (a Glasgow coma scale of less than 8).

National Poisons Information Service

The National Poisons Information Service provides a 24-hour information service on the symptoms and management of poisoning by more than 11 000 drugs, chemicals and plants. At the heart of this service is a computerized database, TOXBASE, and information is provided from regional centres throughout the UK. In addition, some ambulance controls can access TOXBASE.

Centre Telephone numbers
Belfast 02890 240503
Birmingham 0121 507 5588/9
Cardiff 02920 709901
Edinburgh 0131 536 2300
Leeds 0113 243 0715
London 020 7635 9191
Newcastle 0191 232 5131

Severe acute asthma

Deaths from this condition remain distressingly common and many could be prevented. It is important to recognize a patient who is at risk of developing cardiopulmonary arrest; cyanosis, bradycardia and quiet breath sounds (the silent chest) are particularly ominous signs, but appropriate treatment may prevent the inexorable progression to cardiopulmonary arrest. The treatments to be employed in this situation are well described in the standard textbooks of medicine and will not be considered further here.

The treatment of patients with established cardiopulmonary arrest is complicated by high airways resistance that makes ventilation difficult and often ineffective; furthermore, the high pressures required are likely to cause gastric distension and subsequent regurgitation. Tracheal intubation and ventilation with 100% oxygen is the preferred treatment and help from the ambulance service may well be required. Tension pneumothorax must be excluded (it may be the principal cause of the arrest) by comparing the breath sounds on the two sides of the chest and the position of the trachea. If the clinical picture suggests that this is likely, needle thoracocentesis must be performed, or a chest drain inserted. Needle thoracocentesis is performed by inserting a wide bore needle (for example an intravenous cannula), into the second intercostal space on the appropriate side. This procedure should be within the capabilities of any doctor and increasingly paramedics are being trained in the technique. The insertion of a chest drain outside hospital is not unduly difficult – sterile pre-packed units designed for single use are available at relatively modest cost and should be carried by practitioners working as part of an immediate care scheme. Chest drainage is a procedure that is relatively straightforward, undoubtedly life saving in certain situations, yet not at present widely practised outside hospital. It deserves to be far more widely employed.

Not only is ventilation difficult in asthmatics who have suffered cardiopulmonary arrest but chest compression is also hindered by hyperinflation of the chest. Open chest methods of cardiac massage are often recommended but there are obvious practical difficulties with this outside hospital. These patients are usually young and previously healthy, a fact that leads to the most strenuous resuscitation attempts. One can only do one's best and acknowledge the difficulties of resuscitation in this situation, especially outside hospital.

Some patients with severe acute asthma who present with the picture of cardiopulmonary arrest may, in fact, be profoundly bradycardic (before the onset of terminal asystole). Oxygenation is the most important treatment with chest compressions to maintain the circulation; atropine and occasionally external pacing may sometimes help.

Trauma

Practitioners who work as part of an immediate care scheme will often be called by the ambulance service to assist with the management of traumatized patients; in the UK by far the most common cause is road traffic accidents. These doctors will have undertaken special training and this section is not intended to provide this. Any member of the practice team, however, may find themselves assisting in an emergency and, in this section, some important principles behind the management of patients with major trauma are covered, hopefully to provide guidance to the non-specialist in this situation.

Once cardiac arrest has occurred in a victim of trauma at or near the scene of an accident, the outlook is very poor, but not hopeless. It is vital to realize that many such arrests can be prevented by the recognition and treatment of the common complications of trauma. Some modification of the usual techniques of airway management and circulatory support may be required, but the principles behind this are straightforward and their application is not usually complicated.

The principal objective of the management of patients suffering major trauma outside hospital is to stabilize the situation and perform any immediately necessary treatments before the rapid evacuation of the casualty to hospital. Time is the critical factor; the patient needs to be in hospital as soon as possible and only immediately necessary life-saving treatments should be performed at the scene. All too often undue time is wasted trying to gain intravenous access or perform some other manoeuvre of questionable value under very difficult circumstances, when the interest of the patient would be best served by immediate transfer to hospital. Even worse is the situation where well-intentioned health care professionals without any special expertise or training in the management of major trauma feel obliged to stop at an accident and provide assistance, thereby interrupting the work of paramedics who are specifically trained, practised and experienced in managing the common problems that occur in these circumstances.

There are many causes of cardiac arrest in traumatized patients. Penetrating or blunt injury directly affecting the heart is an obvious cause but, in many cases, cardiac arrest occurs as a consequence of hypoxia or hypovalemia complicating multiple injuries – this is often amenable to treatment. Head injury with direct trauma to the brain or following raised intracranial pressure is a further mechanism.

The cardiac rhythm most frequently associated with cardiac arrest following trauma is electromechanical dissociation or asystole; ventricular fibrillation is much less frequent but may occur as a primary rhythm or complicate resuscitation attempts. In most cases the heart itself is relatively healthy and is only rarely responsible for causing the cardiac arrest (unlike most non-traumatized adult cases of cardiac arrest). The priority in these patients is to prevent cardiac arrest from occurring by the prompt recognition and treatment of the complications most likely to cause it. The list of reversible causes contained in the universal algorithm (see Figure 3.4) is particularly important in this regard.

Basic life support

There are often important implications for rescuer safety at the scene of accidents. If in doubt stay out until advice from the emergency services has been obtained. An additional safety issue is the presence of blood or other potentially infected secretions and appropriate precautions should be taken.

If cervical spine injury is suspected from the clinical picture or the mechanism of injury, head tilt should not be performed; the jaw thrust technique will enable basic ventilation in most patients. Both ventilation and chest compressions require considerable care if there are fractures of the chest wall or sternum to prevent further injury occurring. The provision of adequate ventilation is a high priority, taking particular care to avoid gastric distension and possible regurgitation or vomiting. External bleeding must be controlled as a matter of urgency by direct compression of the bleeding point and elevation of the affected limb.

Advanced life support

The provision of high concentration inspired oxygen is vital in all seriously injured patients. For those breathing, spontaneously facemasks with a reservoir bag will suffice. If the patient is unconscious, airway patency should be assured by inserting a Guedel airway. There are fewer restrictions on the use of the Guedel airway than the nasopharyngeal airway; the latter should be used with extreme caution if there is any likelihood of a fracture of the anterior base of the skull, but should be employed if there is no other way of adequately opening the airway.

Tracheal intubation offers many theoretical advantages in the management of the airway in unconscious traumatized patients. If these patients can be intubated without the use of sedative or paralysing drugs, however, their prognosis is exceedingly poor and few survive. Few non-specialists could employ these drugs safely in this situation. Paramedics are not trained to use these agents. There is a lack of published data about the use of the laryngeal mask airway in this situation but it offers several theoretical advantages; it is usually easier to insert than a tracheal tube and visualization of the airway with a laryngoscope is not required. The device might be employed in patients trapped with limited access to the airway and some protection of the airway is provided from the effects of regurgitation or blood or other secretions entering from the oropharynx.

Once ventilation is established careful examination of the chest is mandatory to exclude the presence of a pneumothorax and must be repeated frequently to ensure that a tension pneumothorax is not developing. The venous pressure in the neck should also be monitored to detect the presence of pericardial tamponade as soon as possible, particularly in the presence of electromechanical dissociation. Emergency pericardiocentesis may be life saving and is relatively easy to perform. In a dire emergency a wide bore needle from an intravenous cannula will suffice. These are two relatively common lethal consequences of trauma that can easily be treated provided they are recognized.

Hypovolaemia from blood loss is another potentially correctable consequence of trauma. In the case of external haemorrhage the blood loss will be evident, but it is important to remember that serious internal (concealed) bleeding may also occur. This may follow fractures, particularly of the pelvis and large bones; the ruptured spleen or liver are additional sources.

The traditional management of the victims of trauma who are hypovolaemic has been the rapid infusion of crystalloid fluids through large bore cannulae in quantities sufficient to maintain an adequate systolic blood pressure. The wisdom of this practice has been seriously questioned recently. Several clinical studies have reported an adverse outcome in patients given immediate fluid resuscitation at the scene of trauma compared with patients who received volume replacement in hospital when definitive treatment was possible. It is suggested that the detrimental effect might be due to the dislodgment of clot following the increase in blood pressure that follows infusion of fluid. There is impressive evidence from animal work that aggressive fluid replacement leads to the fibrin plug that had stopped the haemorrhage becoming dislodged when the blood pressure increases. The infusion of fluids available outside hospital serves only to dilute the clotting factors present in blood with the possibility that haemostasis becomes less effective.

In the laboratory, animals resuscitated to a high blood pressure had significantly greater blood loss and higher mortality. Animals resuscitated following a prolonged period of hypotension became acidotic and also faired badly. Those resuscitated to a moderate degree did best in accord with the concept of controlled hypotension. The principle behind hypotensive resuscitation is to provide adequate perfusion to the essential organs, i.e. maintaining an adequate blood pressure to perfuse the heart, brain and kidneys. Higher pressures perfuse organs that might wait until the resuscitation room and has the additional risks outlined above. A systolic blood pressure of around 85 mmHg is thought to be the ideal pressure to achieve this goal and there is an important practical correlate, because the radial pulse becomes palpable at around this pressure.

This debate has some important practical consequences for the primary health care team. In the first place less importance is attached to siting intravenous cannualae and the infusion of large volumes of fluid in shocked patients. Certainly time should not be wasted at the scene trying to site intravenous cannualae under difficult conditions and thereby delay the transport of the patient. Further attempts to gain intravenous access can be made in the ambulance en route to hospital. The maintenance of a palpable radial pulse or a systolic blood pressure of around 85 mmHg would seem a reasonable goal on the basis of current evidence. There are so many variables in the circumstances under discussion that very often decisions can only be made by considering the circumstances of the individual patient. The concepts discussed above also assume that the patient can be rapidly evacuated to hospital, but if the patient is trapped (a relatively common occurrence in road traffic accidents) decisions can only be made in the light of the situation present at the scene.

Electric shock

Injury caused by electric current may occur from a number of sources — from the electric mains, both domestic (240 volts at 50–60 Hz in the UK) or the higher voltages seen in industrial applications. Rarely, injuries from high tension cables on electrical pylons or overhead supplies to railways may be encountered. Lightening strike is another possible cause and may be responsible for injuries to several people in one incident.

Injuries from electricity result from the direct effect of electric current on tissues and from the generation of heat as current passes through the body. The basic mechanisms that result in cardiopulmonary arrest are:

- Arrhythmias caused by the direct action of electricity on the myocardium
- Respiratory arrest from paralysis or tetanic contraction of the diaphragm and chest wall musculature
- Direct effect of electric current causing inhibition of the medullary respiratory centre, again causing primarily a respiratory arrest.

Obviously more than one mechanism may be operative in an individual patient and, as we have seen elsewhere, hypoxic cardiac arrest may follow persistent respiratory arrest. Muscular paralysis may persist for up to 30 minutes after high voltage shocks and respiratory support will be required throughout this time.

There are some important practical considerations relating to the resuscitation of these patients. The first concern is rescuer safety – it is obvious that the power should be turned off before approaching the casualty, but there are traps for the unwary, particularly if high tension cables are involved. High voltages can arc and conduct through the ground surrounding the casualty, particularly under wet conditions. In addition, bird strike is a relatively common occurrence with overground high tension cables and power may be restarted automatically after a brief time interval without the cause of the current leak that automatically shuts off the power having been established.

Basic life support should be carried out according to the usual guidelines having regard for the possibility of cervical spine injury if the casualty has fallen. Burnt or smouldering clothing should be removed to prevent further thermal injury. It is important to secure the airway, preferably by tracheal intubation if possible, as soon as practicable because soft tissue swelling may develop rapidly particularly in patients with burns to the face, mouth or neck. Intravenous fluids will be required in the presence of hypovolaemic shock or if significant soft tissue destruction has occurred. These measures may be initiated before hospital admission, particularly if delay is anticipated in the provision of secondary care.

Ventricular fibrillation or asystole should be treated according to the standard protocols – there is inadequate evidence on which to base special recommendations

Cardiac rhythm disturbance

Bradycardia

Bradycardia is defined rather arbitrarily as a ventricular rate below 60 beats per minute. The rate may be low in absolute terms but it is important to recognize those patients where the rate is too slow for the haemodynamic state of the patient, i.e. when a relative bradycardia is present. Bradycardia may precede cardiopulmonary arrest or complicate the post-resuscitation period and treatment may be successfully undertaken outside hospital. Formal guidelines have been published by the European Resuscitation Council but are detailed and are designed for those treating the condition relatively frequently; the algorithms might be carried in the emergency bag for the time when they are needed. Doctors with an interest in pre-hospital care will be familiar with the algorithm and interested readers will find more details in the references.

Some important principles of the treatment of bradycardia are worth stating. The first of these is that treatment should depend on the haemodynamic status of the patient; precise definition of the arrhythmia matters little as the treatment (usually by drugs like atropine or pacing) does not depend greatly on the cause or precise ECG diagnosis. Oxygen should be administered by a method appropriate to the condition of the patient – if breathing spontaneously via a facemask or nasal prongs. Atropine is the first drug usually employed, the recommended dose being 500 μg intravenously, repeated as necessary to a maximum of 3 mg. If atropine is ineffective, adrenergic drugs should be employed – adrenaline is the one likely to be carried in general practice but isoprenaline is also suitable. It is important to provide effective analgesia in patients who are in pain, e.g. following myocardial infarction, to mitigate the effect of the increased vagal tone that will cause bradycardia in this situation.

If the patient is unconscious, basic life support should be instituted without delay, but occasionally chest percussion may be sufficient to produce a cardiac output. This is performed in a similar manner to the precordial thump but with less force.

It is now possible to pace patients outside hospital by the use of non-invasive transcutaneous pacemakers. Many defibrillators, including some carried by the ambulance service, have the facility to do this by using adhesive defibrillator electrodes to administer the pacing stimulus. The technique is essentially a holding procedure until temporary transvenous pacing can be established in hospital, but it may prove life saving in an emergency and buy time until definitive treatment is available. The chief drawback of this method is discomfort caused by skeletal muscle stimulation and anaesthesia or sedation may be required. Although pacing is an effective method of treating bradycardia it remains an unfortunate fact that it is usually ineffective in the treatment of asystolic cardiac arrest unless some evidence of spontaneous cardiac electrical activity like P waves or QRS complexes is present.

Tachycardia

Tachycardia is said to be present when the ventricular (QRS) rate is 100 beats per minute or more. In this section we are concerned with tachycardias associated with a perfusing rhythm – treatment of pulseless ventricular tachycardia is the same as for ventricular fibrillation as described elsewhere. The correct treatment of many tachyarrhythmias may prevent the progression to cardiac arrest.

As in the case of bradycardia, the European Resuscitation Council has produced guidelines for the management of tachyarrhythmias that precede cardiac arrest or complicate the post-resuscitation period. These are detailed, but difficult for the non-specialist (who may treat the condition very infrequently) to memorize. The algorithms will not be covered in detail in this book and those with an interest in this subject should consult the references. Some general principles of the treatment of tachycardia that do have practical significance for the average GP can be given, however.

It cannot be stated too emphatically that the management of an individual patient with a tachycardia depends on the haemodynamic effects produced by the arrhythmia. Remember that the rate of a tachycardia is not usually the deciding factor in making a decision about treatment. For example a young person with a normal heart may tolerate a ventricular rate in excess of 200 without haemodynamic embarrassment, yet a patient with myocardial impairment (for example from previous infarction) may tolerate a slower tachycardia very poorly.

In most situations outside hospital antiarrhythmic treatment will not be required providing the patient is maintaining an output. Oxygen should be given with appropriate analgesia if required (especially in the case of myocardial infarction), while arrangements are made to transfer the patient urgently to hospital. Standard therapy for heart failure should also be given.

The ECG plays a crucial role in the diagnosis and treatment of tachyarrhythmias and one should always be recorded if the time and condition of the patient permit. Always record a 12-lead ECG and send it with the patient to the receiving hospital as documentation of what may be a transient arrhythmia; it may greatly help the subsequent management of the patient. The effects of carotid sinus massage may also be documented, but caution is necessary with elderly patients who may have atheromatous carotid artery disease.

Classification

Tachycardias may be classified into two categories depending on the width of the QRS complex (narrow or broad complex). A narrow complex tachycardia has a QRS duration of 100 ms (2.5 small squares on the ECG paper) or less, while a broad complex tachycardia will have a QRS duration greater than this. Narrow complex tachycardias are nearly always supraventricular in origin and arise from tissues situated above the bifurcation of the bundle of His. Broad complex tachycardias usually arise below the bifurcation of a bundle of His when they are then described as ventricular. When conduction of a supraventricular tachycardia is delayed (for example by bundle branch block) the QRS complexes will also be broad and the ECG will resemble ventricular tachycardia. In the context of patients with cardiac arrest, however, broad complex tachycardias will nearly always be ventricular in origin and the possibility of the rhythm being a supraventricular one conducted aberrantly can be dismissed. Little harm will come from treating a supraventricular tachycardia as a ventricular one, but the converse (treating a ventricular tachycardia as if it were supraventricular in origin), may be disastrous.

Broad complex tachycardia

Lignocaine is the antiarrhythmic drug likely to be available outside hospital and is currently recommended for the treatment of ventricular tachycardia when the patient is reasonably stable; 50 mg is the recommended dose given over 2 minutes and repeated every 5 minutes (if required) up to a total dose of 200 mg. In the event of successful conversion of the rhythm an infusion at a rate of 2 mg per minute is also recommended. It is doubtful that most patients in this category will need antiarrhythmic drug treatment before transfer to hospital. Nearly all antiarrhythmic drugs have important negative inotropic effects, particularly when used in high doses or in combination. This effect may lead to a worsening in the patient's condition, particularly when conversion of the rhythm does not occur. Antiarrhythmic drugs also have pro-arrhythmic effects particularly when used in combination (and remember a patient may be taking other antiarrhythmic drugs orally on a chronic basis).

Where adverse clinical signs accompany ventricular tachycardia (a systolic blood pressure less than 90 mmHg, a pulse rate greater than 150 or heart failure or chest pain), the current guidelines recommend sedation and DC cardioversion, but the circumstances where this would be a practical proposition outside hospital must be very limited. Other recommended antiarrhythmic agents like flecanide, bretylium and amiodarone are unlikely to be available outside hospital, and amiodarone should given by a central venous line. The treatment of most patients outside hospital should centre on optimizing oxygenation, controlling chest pain with nitrates and opiates and treating heart failure with opiates, diuretics and nitrates while arranging urgent transport to hospital.

Narrow complex tachycardias

Patients with a narrow complex tachycardia are seen occasionally in general practice. They may have a history of previous attacks and some will be known to have the Wolff-Parkinson-White syndrome. As with all tachycardias, oxygen should be given and an ECG should be recorded if the patient's condition allows. Vagotonic procedures are the initial treatment and should then be performed with the ECG running whenever possible. Coughing, the Valsava manoeuvre or splashing the face with cold water are worth trying before proceeding to carotid sinus massage. These patients are often young and the possibility of carotid artery disease need not be considered; in older patients, particularly those with a bruit, there is some risk of rupturing an atheromatus plaque which may embolize into the cerebral circulation resulting in a stroke.

Adenosine is the drug of choice if vagotonic procedures are unsuccessful. It has the advantage of having an extremely short half-life (10–15 s) and negative inotropic effects are not a problem in practice. The drug needs ideally to be given rapidly into a fast running intravenous infusion and flushed in. An initial dose of 3 mg is recommended followed by 6 mg and subsequently 12 mg if necessary. Transient nausea, flushing and chest discomfort may occur but are usually very short-lived phenomena. The author has employed this drug on several occasions outside hospital, but it should be pointed out that he does so with full resuscitation equipment including a defibrillator available – precautions that are necessary during any attempt to treat arrhythmias, especially outside hospital. As with broad complex tachycardia, the most important treatments before hospitalization are the provision of oxygen and the treatment of anxiety or heart failure while arranging urgent admission.

References and further reading

Chamberlain DA (1997) Periarrest arrhythmias. *Br J Anaesthesia*, **79**:198–202.

Colquhoun MC, Vincent R (1999) Management of the periarrest arrhythmias. In *ABC of Resuscitation*, 4th edn (Colquhoun MC, Handley AJ, Evans TR, eds). pp 14–18. BMJ Books, London.

European Resuscitation Council (1998) Periarrest arrhythmias: management of arrhythmias associated with cardiac arrest. In *European Resuscitation Council Guidelines for Resuscitation*. Elsevier, Oxford.

Greaves I, Hodgetts T, Porter K (1997) *Emergency care: a textbook for paramedics*. WB Sanders, London.

Harries M (1999) Near drowning. In *ABC of Resuscitation*, 4th edn (Colquhoun MC, Handley AJ, Evans TR, eds). pp 49–51. BMJ Books, London.

International Liaison Committee on Resuscitation (1997) Special resuscitation situations. An advisory statement on conditions which may require modification of techniques. *Resuscitation*, **34**:129–49.

Jones AL (1998) Initial management of poisoned patients in the out of hospital environment. *Pre-hospital Immediate Care*, **2**:141–9.

Robertson C, Redman AD (1995) *The Management of Major Trauma*. Oxford University Press, Oxford.

Skinner D, Swain A, Peyton R, Robertson C (eds) (1997) *Cambridge Textbook of Accident and Emergency Medicine*. Cambridge University Press, Cambridge.

Skinner D, Driscoll P, Earlham R (1998) *ABC of Major Trauma*. BMJ Books, London.

Chapter 6

Anaphylaxis

Anaphylaxis is a life-threatening medical emergency requiring rapid diagnosis and the correct medical treatment if cardiorespiratory arrest is to be prevented. So important is the correct management of anaphylaxis that a multidisciplinary project team of the Resuscitation Council (UK) was established to formulate guidelines on the optimal management of the condition. These were published in June 1999, and the recommendations in this chapter are largely based on the report of this project team.

Anaphylactic reactions may follow exposure to a variety of substances with insect stings, drugs, and certain foods, particularly nuts, being the most common. Anaphylaxis to any of these may be encountered in general practice, and the possibility of anaphylaxis following immunization must always been borne in mind. Practice protocols should exist for its management and the facilities to treat the condition appropriately must be readily available wherever immunizations or other injections are performed.

Clinical picture

Anaphylactic reactions usually present clinically with angioneurotic oedema, urticaria, dyspnoea and hypotension. Other symptoms include rhinitis, conjunctivitis, abdominal pain, diarrhoea and vomiting. Patients sometimes experience a feeling of impending doom. The extent of the individual symptoms varies between cases and some patients may succumb to irreversible asthma or laryngeal oedema in the absence of the more generalized features described above. Cardiovascular collapse is common and is caused by widespread vasodilation with loss of plasma volume from the circulation. Reactions may vary greatly in severity and speed of onset; symptoms usually occur rapidly following intravenous injections and some insect stings, but may develop more slowly in other circumstances with resultant diagnostic difficulty.

A full history and clinical examination should be undertaken as far as

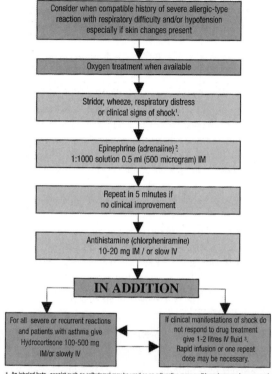

Anaphylactic Reactions for Adults
Treatment by First Medical Responders

Consider when compatible history of severe allergic-type reaction with respiratory difficulty and/or hypotension especially if skin changes present

↓

Oxygen treatment when available

↓

Stridor, wheeze, respiratory distress or clinical signs of shock[1].

↓

Epinephrine (adrenaline)[2]
1:1000 solution 0.5 ml (500 microgram) IM

↓

Repeat in 5 minutes if no clinical improvement

↓

Antihistamine (chlorpheniramine)
10-20 mg IM / or slow IV

↓

IN ADDITION

For all severe or recurrent reactions and patients with asthma give Hydrocortisone 100-500 mg IM/or slowly IV

If clinical manifestations of shock do not respond to drug treatment give 1-2 litres IV fluid [3]. Rapid infusion or one repeat dose may be necessary.

1. An inhaled beta₂-agonist such as salbutamol may be used as an adjunctive measure if bronchospasm is severe and does not respond rapidly to other treatment.
2. If profound shock is judged **immediately** life threatening give CPR/ALS if necessary. Consider **slow** intravenous epinephrine (adrenaline) 1:10,000 solution. This is **hazardous** and is recommended only for an experienced practitioner who can also obtain IV access without delay.
Note the different strength of epinephrine (adrenaline) that may be required for IV use.
3. A crystalloid may be safer than a colloid.

IM = intramuscular

Published with kind permission of the BMJ Publishing Group in conjunction with the Resuscitation Council (UK)

AURUM   Resuscitation Council (UK)

Supplied as a service to the healthcare profession by AURUM PHARMACEUTICALS LTD

Journal of Accident and Emergency Medicine 1999: 16(4)243-247
A report on the Emergency Medical Treatment of Anaphylactic Reactions
by a Project Team of the Resuscitation Council (UK)

Figure 6.1 The management of anaphylaxis in adults (Aurum and Resuscitation Council UK)

Anaphylactic Reactions for Children
Treatment by First Medical Responders

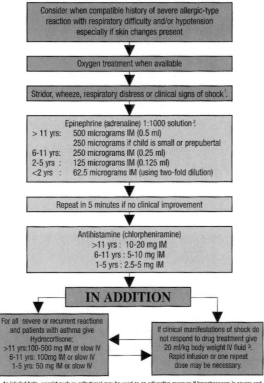

Consider when compatible history of severe allergic-type reaction with respiratory difficulty and/or hypotension especially if skin changes present

Oxygen treatment when available

Stridor, wheeze, respiratory distress or clinical signs of shock[1].

Epinephrine (adrenaline) 1:1000 solution[2]
> 11 yrs: 500 micrograms IM (0.5 ml)
            250 micrograms if child is small or prepubertal
6-11 yrs: 250 micrograms IM (0.25 ml)
2-5 yrs : 125 micrograms IM (0.125 ml)
<2 yrs : 62.5 micrograms IM (using two-fold dilution)

Repeat in 5 minutes if no clinical improvement

Antihistamine (chlorpheniramine)
>11 yrs : 10-20 mg IM
6-11 yrs : 5-10 mg IM
1-5 yrs : 2.5-5 mg IM

IN ADDITION

For all severe or recurrent reactions and patients with asthma give Hydrocortisone:
>11 yrs:100-500 mg IM or slow IV
6-11 yrs: 100mg IM or slow IV
1-5 yrs: 50 mg IM or slow IV

If clinical manifestations of shock do not respond to drug treatment give 20 ml/kg body weight IV fluid[3]. Rapid infusion or one repeat dose may be necessary.

1. An inhaled beta$_2$-agonist such as salbutamol may be used as an adjunctive measure if bronchospasm is severe and does not respond rapidly to other treatment.
2. If profound shock is judged **immediately** life threatening give CPR/ALS if necessary. Consider **slow** intravenous epinephrine (adrenaline) 1:10,000 solution. This is **hazardous** and is recommended only for an experienced practitioner who can also obtain IV access without delay.
Note the different strength of epinephrine (adrenaline) that may be required for IV use.
3. A crystalloid may be safer than a colloid.

IM = intramuscular

**Published with kind permission of the BMJ Publishing Group
in conjunction with the Resuscitation Council (UK)**

🏛 AURUM   💚 Resuscitation Council (UK)

Supplied as a service to the healthcare profession by AURUM PHARMACEUTICALS LTD

*Journal of Accident and Emergency Medicine 1999; 16(4)243-247
A report on the Emergency Medical Treatment of Anaphylactic Reactions
by a Project Team of the Resuscitation Council (UK)*

Figure 6.2 The management of anaphylaxis in children (Aurum and Resuscitation Council UK)

circumstances permit. A history of previous allergic reactions and recent exposure to a possible cause are the crucial features of the history. A second attack of anaphylaxis is by no means invariable with a repeated challenge (for example with penicillin), and approximately only one-half of patients remain vulnerable after repeated exposure to insect stings. Peanuts and some food allergies may result in a persistent susceptibility after a first attack, but eventual resolution has been described.

Treatment

No definitive clinical trial evidence exists on which to base guidelines for the treatment of anaphylaxis, and it is unlikely that any will be produced. These guidelines are therefore based on the considerable clinical experience that exists with the management of the condition. The project group recognized two main problems with the treatment of anaphylaxis in most situations in which it occurs:

- adrenaline (epinephrine) is greatly underused and treatment with chlorpheniramine (Piriton) and hydrocortisone has more frequently been given instead
- adrenaline has often been given intravenously, especially by paramedics and in A & E Departments, when it should be given intramuscularly.

All patients should recline in a position of comfort. Lying the patient flat and elevating the legs may be helpful in the present of hypotension but may aggravate breathing difficulties. Oxygen should be administered at a high flow rate with a delivery system that ensures a concentration of inspired oxygen approaching 100%.

Adrenaline

Adrenaline is generally agreed to be the most important drug for any severe anaphylactic reaction. Its alpha adrenergic agonist activity reverses the peripheral vasodilation that leads to the formation of angioneurotic oedema. Its beta adrenoceptor stimulating activity dilates the airways, has positive inotropic actions and suppresses the release of mediators of anaphylaxis like histamine and leukotrienes. The earlier it is given after the onset of a reaction the better and when given intramuscularly is very safe –

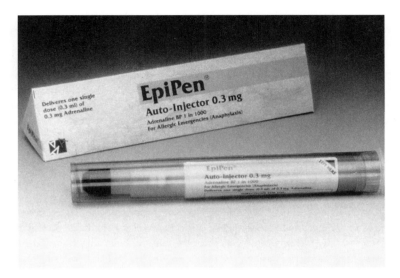

Figure 6.3 Epipen

serious cardiac arrhythmias may follow intravenous administration. Absorption is too slow and unpredictable with subcutaneous injection and this route should be abandoned.

Adrenaline should be administered intramuscularly to all patients with clinical signs of shock, airway swelling or definite difficulties in breathing. It is rapidly absorbed and for adults a dose of 500 μg (0.5 ml of 1 : 1000 solution) should be administered intramuscularly and this dose should be repeated after about 5 minutes in the absence of clinical improvement or if deterioration occurs. In some cases several doses may be required, particularly in the presence of hypotension or if improvement is only transient and followed by later deterioration.

The doses of adrenaline recommended for children are:

- > 11 years: up to 500 μg IM (0.5 ml 1 : 1000 solution)
- 6–11 years: 250 μg IM (0.25 ml 1 : 1000 solution)
- 2–5 years: 125 μg IM (0.125 ml 1 : 1000 solution)
- < 2 years: 62.5 μg IM.

As with adults repeated doses may be necessary.

Devices exist that enable patients to inject themselves with adrenaline when exposure to a known allergen, for example bee stings, occurs, enabling the drug to be given before medical help is available.

Intravenous adrenaline is potentially hazardous and is reserved for the treatment of patients with profound shock that is life threatening. Diluted to at least 1 : 10 000, intravenous injection should be given slowly with continuous monitoring of the electrocardiogram. A further dilution of adrenaline (for example to 1 : 100 000) may be safer for the intravenous route.

Antihistamines

An antihistamine should be administered, and chlorpheniramine (Piriton) is the agent most widely available in general practice. The drug should be given by slow intravenous infusion or by intramuscular injection. Dose is determined by age:

- Adults and children over 11 years: 10–20 mg IM
- Children 6–11 years: 5–10 mg IM
- Children 1–5 years: 2.5–5 mg IM.

Hydrocortisone

Hydrocortisone should be administered and may help avert later consequences, particularly in asthmatics. The drug should be given by slow intravenous infusion but may be given by the intramuscular route. The dose is determined by age as follows:

- Adults and children over 11 years of age: 100–500 mg
- Children 6–11 years: 100 mg
- Children 1–5 years: 50 mg.

Other treatment

If severe hypotension does not respond rapidly to the treatments already described, intravenous infusion of fluids should be employed. Crystalloids are recommended and a rapid infusion of 1–2 litres may be needed in adults. Children should receive 20 ml/kg of body weight and the dose repeated if there is no adequate response. Nebulized beta agonists, such as salbutamol, may be useful, particularly when bronchospasm is a major feature of the reaction and does not respond rapidly to the other treatments employed. Adrenaline may also be given via a nebulizer and is occasionally employed.

Follow-up

Patients with a significant anaphylactic reaction should be warned of the possibility of a recurrence of symptoms after initial successful treatment and in most circumstances should be admitted to hospital and kept under observation until the risk has passed. This precaution is particularly important when the onset of a reaction is slow or when the provoking agent is unknown. Reactions occurring in asthmatics or where asthma is a major feature of the reaction, deserve particular supervision after initial treatment. Where the possibility of continuing absorption of antigen exists or in patients with a history of a biphasic reaction during a previous episode, prolonged surveillance will be required. All victims should be advised to wear a bracelet or necklace that will inform bystanders of their propensity to anaphylactic reactions in the event of a future attack. Precautions should obviously be taken as far as practical, to avoid subsequent exposure. Investigation in a specialist allergy clinic is recommended in patients with severe reactions and may prove particularly important in those where the allergen is not identified at the time of the attack.

References and further reading

Ewen PW (1997) Treatment of anaphylactic reactions. *Prescribers Journal*, **37**:125–32.
Ewen PW (1998) Anaphylaxis. *Br Med J*, **316**:1442–5.
Project Team of the Resuscitation Council (UK) (1999) The emergency medical treatment of anaphylactic reactions. *Br J Accident Emergency Med*, **16**:243–7.
Statement from Resuscitation Council (UK) and the Joint Royal Colleges Ambulance Service Liaison Committee (1997) The use of adrenaline for anaphylactic shock (for Ambulance paramedics). *Ambulance UK*, **12**:16.

Chapter 7

Resuscitation of infants and children

Introduction

Fortunately it is very rare for members of the primary health care team to attempt the resuscitation of infants and children. Life-threatening emergencies do occur in this age group however, and the actions of those present will greatly influence the chances of a full recovery. For this reason alone we include this chapter, but of equal importance is our basic philosophy – that by careful management of the sick child, particularly with regard to the maintenance of the airway and providing adequate ventilation, many cases of cardiopulmonary arrest may be prevented.

There is a fundamental difference in the approach to the resuscitation of children and infants compared to adults. The resuscitation of adult victims of cardiac arrest is based on the observation that the great majority are of primarily cardiac origin often occurring with little or no warning and due to cardiac rhythm disturbance, most frequently ventricular fibrillation. The rapid application of a defibrillatory countershock is the key to success.

A cardiac arrest due primarily to cardiac disease is rare in infants and children, and ventricular fibrillation or tachycardia are rarely seen. The primary cause of cardiopulmonary arrest in this age group is usually respiratory failure, which leads ultimately to bradycardia and asystolic cardiac arrest if not recognized and treated. Cardiac arrest is the end stage of a progressive sequence of events and many deaths could be prevented by the early recognition and treatment of the seriously ill child. The prognosis for infants and children who do experience cardiac arrest is very poor indeed with survival rates of between and 3% and 17% having been reported in hospital series, with many survivors showing residual neurological impairment. Most of the reported series are small, and the difference in success rate depends on many factors, including the underlying cause (a primarily respiratory cause has a better prognosis than a primarily cardiac one) and the location of the arrest (cardiac arrest occurring outside hospital has a worse prognosis).

With children, the prevention and early recognition of a condition that may lead to respiratory collapse is the priority; aggressive treatment at this stage may prevent the inevitable progression to cardiac arrest. The challenge for those working in primary care is to recognize children who are potentially seriously ill at the earliest possible stage, hopefully before respiration is compromised. This challenge is formidable, as many potentially serious illnesses have non-specific symptoms in their early stages (meningococcal disease) or deterioration may occur rapidly with little initial indication of the underlying seriousness of the child's condition (epiglottitis). Children and infants with difficulty breathing obviously require detailed assessment with examination directed towards the adequacy of ventilation and oxygenation. Evidence of circulatory compromise is particularly ominous in this situation and requires further intervention to be undertaken as a matter of urgency.

There are many potentially life-threatening medical emergencies in children that may progress to a stage where cardiopulmonary resuscitation is required and their assessment is outside the scope of this book – the reader should consult the standard textbooks of paediatrics.

Paediatric basic life support

In the following discussion the term 'infant' is applied to the child under the age of 1 year, while a child is defined as being between one and eight years of age. Children over the age of eight will still be treated in the same way as younger children but different methods of chest compression may be employed. The sequence of action recommended is summarized in the algorithm (Figure 7.1). As in the case of adult resuscitation it is imperative to check the safety of both rescuer and casualty before starting resuscitation procedures. Assuming no dangers exist, the first stage is to assess responsiveness. Gentle but firm stimulation should be applied while asking 'are you alright?' Children should not be shaken vigorously and if spinal injury is suspected, particularly of the cervical spine, no movement of the child should be induced or permitted. If there is a response, leave the child in the same position provided he is stable and safe. Carry out a more detailed assessment and get help if needed, reassessing the situation as required. If the child does not respond shout for help and start the usual ABC sequence (Airway, Breathing and Circulation).

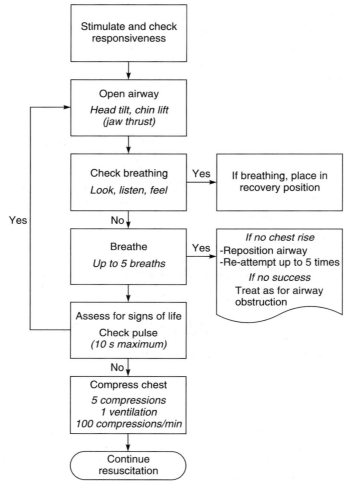

Figure 7.1 European Resuscitation Council Algorithm for Paediatric Basic Life Support © ERC 1999 (from *European Resuscitation Council Guidelines for Resuscitation*, edited by L. Bossaert, 1998, Elsevier, Oxford by kind permission)

Airway

The tongue is the most common cause of airway obstruction in both children and adults, and the head tilt, chin lift procedure is usually adequate to establish airway patency (Figure 7.2). Attempt this procedure if possible in the position in which you find the casualty, placing one hand on the forehead, tilting the head backwards, while simultaneously lifting the chin with your finger tips placed at the point of the chin. It is important not to push on the soft tissues under the chin while doing this. If this proves difficult turn the child on his back and repeat the procedure. The head tilt manoeuvres should be avoided if cervical spine injury is a possibility and in this case the jaw thrust manoeuvre should be employed.

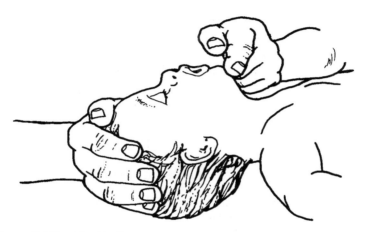

Figure 7.2 Head tilt, chin lift to open an infant's airway

Breathing

Having opened the airway, look, listen and feel for breathing for up to 10 seconds before deciding that breathing is absent. If the child is breathing, place in the recovery position and ensure that breathing continues. If the child is not breathing, carefully remove any obvious obstruction to the airway and give up to five rescue breaths, each of which should cause the chest to rise. With expired air ventilation in the infant, the mouth and nose should be covered by the rescuer's mouth ensuring a good seal (Figure 7.3). Inflation should be carried out steadily over 1–1.5 seconds, sufficient to make the chest visibly rise. Maintaining the head tilt, chin lift position the rescuer's mouth is then removed, watching the chest fall as air is exhaled. For a child the nose should be pinched closed and conventional mouth-to-mouth ventilation should be given again, with each chest inflation occupying 1–1.5 seconds.

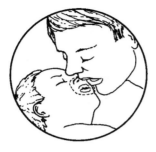

Figure 7.3 Ventilation in an infant: the rescuer's mouth should cover the infant's nose and mouth, ensuring a good seal

If there is difficulty in achieving chest inflation the airway may be obstructed, so open the child's mouth and remove any obstructions. Check that there is adequate head tilt and chin lift and ensure that the neck is not hyperextended. Make up to five attempts to achieve at least two effective chest inflations but if unsuccessful (or if the child is making respiratory movements but no passage of air can be felt or heard), foreign body obstruction of the airway may be present. Treatment of this is described below.

Circulation

Check for the presence of a pulse – in an infant feel for the brachial pulse on the inner aspect of the upper arm (Figure 7.4), while in an older child feel for the carotid pulse in the neck. Check for other signs of a circulation, like movement, swallowing or breathing (more than the occasional gasp), taking no longer than 10 seconds to do this. If signs of a circulation are present, continue rescue breathing if required until the child is breathing effectively on his own. Once this occurs place an unconscious child in the recovery position.

If there are no signs of a circulation or you are unsure (or in infants the pulse is less than 60 beats per minute), start chest compressions and combine them with rescue breaths. For an infant, place the tips of index and middle fingers of one hand on the sternum, one finger's breath below an imaginary line joining the infant's nipples (Figure 7.5). Press down on the sternum with the tips of the fingers to depress it one-third the depth of the infant's chest. Release the pressure and repeat to achieve a rate of 100 compressions per minute. After five compressions a breath is administered and the sequence of five compressions to one breath is continued.

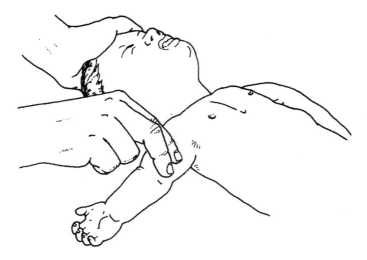

Figure 7.4 Pulse check in an infant – feel for the brachial pulse on the inner aspect of the upper arm for 10 seconds

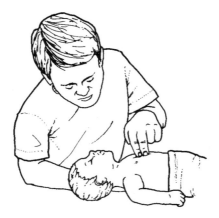

Figure 7.5 Chest compressions in an infant: two fingers on the sternum, one finger's breadth below an imaginary line joining the two nipples

To perform chest compressions in a child, place the heel of one hand over the lower half of the sternum ensuring that you do not compress to the side of, or below the sternum. Lift the fingers to ensure that pressure is not applied over the child's ribs or costal cartilages. Position yourself vertically above the chest and with arms straight compress the sternum one-third the depth of the thorax (Figure 7.6). As with infants, a rate of 100 compressions per minute is employed with a ratio of five compressions to one breath.

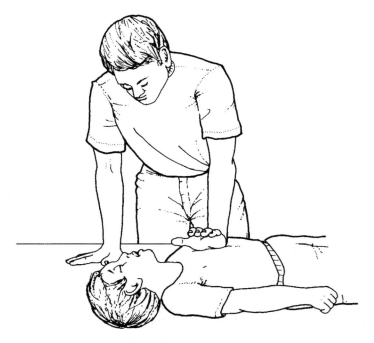

Figure 7.6 Chest compressions in a child: heel of one hand on the lower half of the sternum

In children over the age of approximately 8 years, it may be more appropriate to use the adult two-handed technique to achieve an adequate depth of chest compressions. The heel of one hand is placed over the lower half of the sternum and the other is placed on top. The fingers are interlocked and lifted clear of the rib cage. As with the younger child, the rescuer is positioned vertically above the chest and with arms straight depresses the sternum one-third of the depth of the child's chest. Again, a rate of 100 per minute should be employed but in this situation the ratio of 15 compressions to two breaths ratio, as used in adults, should be employed.

Calling for help

In general practice the procedure for summoning help (and its timing) would depend to some extent on the nature of the emergency and the skill of the rescuers. In most cases, however, it would be best to summon an ambulance when the emergency is first recognized. This may be possible with information received before the doctor arrives so that a dual response from both doctor and ambulance service takes place. In other circumstances, it will usually be most appropriate to send a parent or other carer to summon help while initiating resuscitation. If the rescuer is alone, the usual recommendation is that resuscitation should be performed for about 1 minute before seeking assistance, but the decision must be made in the light of the individual circumstances. It may sometimes be possible to carry an infant or small child to the phone and continue resuscitation.

The obstructed airway: the treatment of choking

If a child is breathing spontaneously, its own efforts to clear the obstruction should be encouraged and intervention should only be attempted if these are ineffective and breathing becomes inadequate. Blind finger sweeps of the mouth are not recommended as these may force a foreign body further into the airway or cause soft tissue damage. The aim of treatment is to create a sharp increase in intrathoracic pressure; the procedures recommended are back blows and chest thrusts.

To perform back blows hold the child prone if possible, with the head lower than the chest and deliver five smart blows to the middle of the back between the shoulder blades. This should be attempted five times and if the procedure fails to dislodge the foreign body, proceed to chest thrusts. Place the child in the supine position and administer five chest thrusts to the sternum in a position similar to that used for chest compressions. Chest thrusts should be sharper and more vigorous than chest compressions and carried out at a rate of about 20 per minute. After the sequence of five back blows and five chest thrusts, the mouth should be examined and any visible foreign bodies removed. Thereafter open the airway and reassess breathing — if this is now present place the child in the recovery position and maintain careful observations. If the child is not breathing attempt five further rescue breaths — if the child is apnoeic or the airway is partially cleared effective ventilation may now be possible. If the airway remains obstructed repeat the cycle but chest thrusts should be used instead of abdominal thrusts after the second sequence of back blows. Subsequently five back blows combined with five chest thrusts or abdominal thrusts in alternate cycles are employed until the airway is cleared. After each cycle of abdominal thrusts (or in an infant chest thrusts) the mouth should be checked, the airway opened and further attempts made to provide rescue breaths.

Abdominal thrusts are performed with the child in the upright position if the child is conscious, but an unconscious child should be laid supine. With the heel of one hand placed in the middle of the upper abdomen, up to five sharp thrusts should be directed upwards towards the diaphragm. Abdominal thrusts are not recommended in infants because severe damage to abdominal viscera may result.

Paediatric advanced life support

Equipment

The practice of advanced life support requires the use of special equipment and often drugs. There are problems with the use of such equipment because a wide range of sizes must be available to correspond with the child or infant requiring resuscitation and the operator must be skilled in their selection and use. This poses obvious practical problems to members of the primary health care team who attempt resuscitation of infants and children very infrequently; it is difficult to maintain the equipment in a state of constant readiness and remain skilled and practised in its use.

Airway

Management of the airway and the provision of ventilation are of prime importance in paediatric resuscitation and respiratory depression is usually the cause of cardiopulmonary arrest. Access to the airway must be provided as soon as possible and the infant or child should be ventilated with as high a concentration of inspired oxygen as possible. The bag/valve/mask device with a suitable oxygen reservoir will enable this, used with a facemask of the appropriate size for the casualty. The mask should be made of clear material and ensure a good seal on the child's face. Circular masks are recommended, particularly when the rescuer is inexperienced (Figure 7.7). The self-inflating bag/valve/mask (Figure 7.8) should incorporate a pressure limited escape valve to prevent a maximum airway pressure of 30–35 cm of

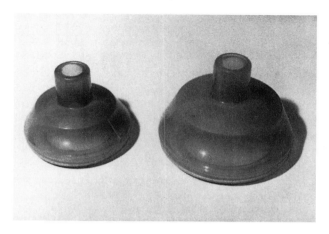

Figure 7.7 Paediatric circular masks

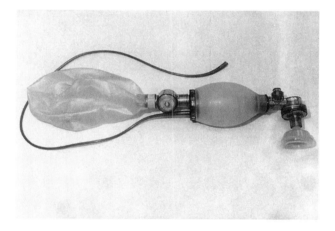

Figure 7.8 Paediatric bag/valve/mask device

water being exceeded. This is necessary to minimize the risk of damage to the lungs by excessive pressure. Bag/valve/mask devices require considerable skill to be used successfully by a single operator and it is usually best considered a two-operator technique. One rescuer controlling the airway and applying the facemask, while the other inflates the bag. A Guedel airway may be inserted if the airway cannot be maintained by correct positioning alone; again a range of sizes will be required in the emergency bag; the correct size is chosen to correspond to the distance from the centre of the mouth to the angle of the jaw.

Expired air ventilation may be also be provided through a facemask. The ubiquitous Laerdal pocket mask would be suitable for older children, and when turned through 180 degrees will fit babies and small children. Models which allow the provision of supplemental oxygen through a side port are available and are strongly recommended.

Tracheal intubation is the ideal method to control the airway; it provides access for efficient ventilation and minimizes the risk of aspiration of gastric contents. Intubation must be achieved rapidly without a prolonged delay in providing basic life support. The technique requires training, and practice is required to maintain proficiency. There are important differences in the anatomy of the larynx of paediatric subjects which necessitate modification of the technique used in adults. A straight-bladed laryngoscope is usually preferred and plain plastic tracheal tubes (Figure 7.9) without an inflatable bulb at the distal end should be employed. The approximate size of the tube for children over one year old can be calculated from the formula:

$$\text{internal diameter (mm)} = \frac{\text{age in years}}{4} + 4$$

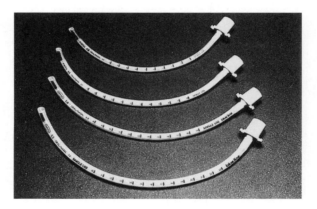

Figure 7.9 Selection of uncuffed tracheal tubes

Most GPs will have neither the training nor the equipment to undertake tracheal intubation and the priority will usually be to establish ventilation via a facemask. Similar considerations apply to the use of the laryngeal mask airway. Appropriately sized laryngeal masks are available for infants and children but their effectiveness in paediatric resuscitation has not yet been established. They are relatively expensive but a range of sizes would be required.

Paramedics in the UK are taught the techniques of intubation in paediatric subjects, which is an additional advantage of summoning the ambulance at an early stage. It is obviously important for members of the primary health care team to be aware of the principles of the technique to work effectively with the ambulance service.

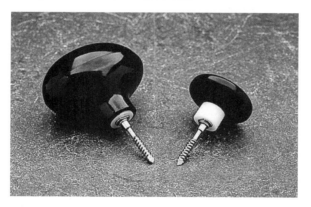

Figure 7.10 Intraosseous needles (Cook Critical Care)

Circulation

Access to the venous circulation is required for the administration of both fluids and drugs, but peripheral venous cannulation is difficult in paediatric subjects, especially when collapsed. Central venous catherization is also difficult and many potentially serious complications may result. It should only be undertaken by appropriately trained, experienced practitioners; this will restrict its use by the primary health care team. The intraosseous route provides a practical alternative, however. The bone marrow of the tibia consists of a venous plexus which drains directly into the central circulation. A special intraosseous cannula or needle (Figure 7.10) is inserted into the tibia to allow the administration of intravenous fluids and even blood; entry into the venous circulation is rapid. Once again special equipment is required but this is relatively inexpensive and one size of needle is appropriate for all age groups. The technique is relatively easy to learn and does not require extensive training or practice (Figure 7.11).

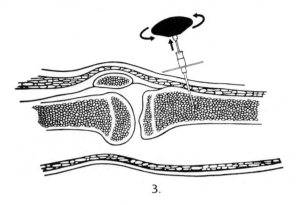

3.

Figure 7.11 Insertion of intraosseous needle

Drug administration

The intravenous and intraosseous routes provide the most certain and reliable routes if access can be established. Drugs may be administered by the tracheal route if an endotracheal tube is in place, and may be the only available route if intravenous or intraosseous access cannot be established. Both adrenaline and atropine may be given by the endobronchial route and should be diluted in the suitable volume of saline and ideally given through a special cannula that reaches just beyond the distal opening of the tracheal tube. There has been inadequate research on this method of drug administration in children. Do recommend precise doses of drugs and their dilution.

Drug doses

It is impractical for personnel who undertake paediatric resuscitation infrequently to memorize the dosage of the drugs that might be required. The Oakley chart employs a length, weight, age nomogram to calculate the appropriate dose of a drug. It is highly recommended that a copy of this or other such guide is carried at all times in the emergency bag.

THE WALSALL PAEDIATRIC RESUSCITATION CHART

NB. ALL DRUG DOSES ARE IN MILLILITRES (MLS), I/V OR INTRAOSSEOUS UNLESS OTHERWISE STATED.

AGE		MONTHS			YEARS				
		3	6	1	3.5	6	10	13	14
WEIGHT (KG)		5	7	10	15	20	30	40	50

ADRENALINE/ 1:10,000 EPINEPHERINE	Initial	0.5	0.7	1	1.5	2	3	4	5
ADRENALINE/ 1:1,000 EPINEPHERINE	Subsequent or initial endotracheal	0.5	0.7	1	1.5	2	3	4	5
SODIUM BICARBONATE 4.2%		10	14	20	30	40	60	80	100
CALCIUM CHLORIDE 10%		0.5	0.7	1	1.5	2	3	4	5
DEXTROSE 10%		25	35	50	75	100	150	200	250
LIGNOCAINE/LIDOCAINE 1%		0.5	0.7	1	1.5	2	3	4	5
INITIAL FLUID BOLUS IN SHOCK		100	140	200	300	400	600	800	1000
ET TUBE SIZE (MM) (Internal diameter)		3.5	4	4	5	6	6.5	7.5	7.5
ET TUBE SIZE (CM) (Length)		10	11	12	14	16	17	18	19
INITIAL DC DEFIBRILLATION (J)		10	15	20	30	40	60	80	100

References:

1. Burke DP, Bowden DF (1993)   Modified Paediatric Resuscitation Chart   BMJ 306:1096-82.

2. ERC (1998)   The 1998 European Resuscitation Council
                                 Guidelines for Paediatric Life Support Sequence
                                 of Actions in European Resuscitation Council
                                 Guidelines for Resuscitation   Elsevier, Oxford P83-97

For further copies of this chart please contact:
Phil Jevon, Resuscitation Training Officer, Manor Hospital, Walsall. WS2 9PS

🏛 AURUM

Supplied as a service to the CPR healthcare profession by AURUM PHARMACEUTICALS LTD

Figure 7.12 Paediatric Resuscitation Chart (Walsall Hospitals NHS Trust)

An alternative method of determining drug doses relies on the length of the child and, while accurate, requires the use of a specially designed tape measure (the Broselow tape).

Management protocols

The first priority in the resuscitation of children is to establish control of the airway and provide effective ventilation preferably with a high concentration of inspired oxygen; subsequent management depends upon the cardiac rhythm. This would usually be monitored through the electrodes of a defibrillator and subsequent treatment depends on whether ventricular fibrillation/ventricular tachycardia is present or whether a non-VF/VT rhythm is found. The latter include asystole and electromechanical dissociation, which are by far the most common finding in infancy and childhood. The algorithm (Figure 7.13) has many similarities to the algorithm used in the resuscitation of adults, with emphasis placed on the early recognition of the cardiac rhythm responsible for arrest.

Check for the pulse in the carotid artery in the neck in a child or, in an infant, on the brachial artery on the inner aspect of the upper arm. No more than 10 seconds should be taken to perform the pulse check. Depending on the findings, the algorithms follows one of two routes.

Non-ventricular fibrillation/tachycardia rhythms

Asystole
Asystole is the most common rhythm seen in paediatric subjects, regardless of whether the cause is respiratory or circulatory. The diagnosis is made from characteristic ECG appearance in a patient with the features of cardiopulmonary arrest. Ensure the correct position of the ECG electrodes, electrical connections and gain on the monitor before diagnosing asystole. Adrenaline (epinephrine) should be administered in a dose of 10 μg per kilogram if intravenous or intraosseous access has been established. The recommended dose for endotracheal administration is 100 μg per kilogram. This should be followed by 3 minutes of basic life support and if asystole persists the dose should be repeated. The cycle of adrenaline followed by 3 minutes of basic life support should be repeated as long as it is thought that continued resuscitation efforts are appropriate or until the rhythm changes. A search for potentially reversible causes should be made between the

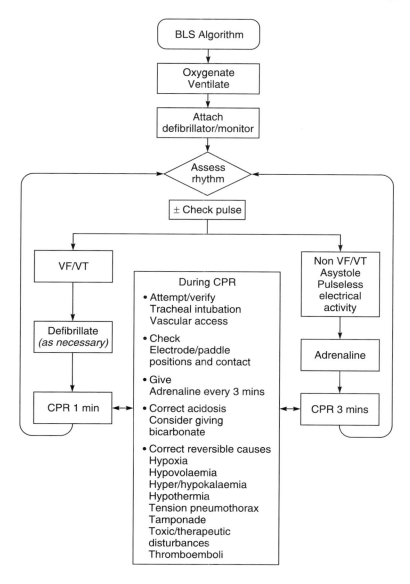

Figure 7.13 European Resuscitation Council algorithm for paediatric advanced life support © ERC 1999 (from *European Resuscitation Council Guidelines for Resuscitation*, edited by L. Bossaert, 1998, Elsevier, Oxford by kind permission)

cycles of CPR. The most important causes are the four Hs (hypoxia, hypovolaemia, hyper/hypokalaemia, hypothermia) and the four Ts (tension pneumothorax, cardiac tamponade, thromboembolic disturbance, toxins and drug overdose).

Alkalizing agents are of unproven benefits and are usually administered in the light of blood gas analysis; there is practically no indication for their use outside hospital.

When hypovolaemia is suspected, an infusion of fluid should be given – 20 ml per kilogram of crystalloid (normal saline or Ringers lactate should be administered).

Electromechanical dissociation (EMD)

This condition is diagnosed in a patient with the clinical picture of cardiopulmonary arrest, but with an ECG that would normally be associated with a cardiac output. If untreated the rhythm will degenerate into bradycardia and asystole. It is managed in the same way as asystole with particular emphasis on the search for (and correction of) reversible causes.

Ventricular fibrillation/pulseless ventricular tachycardia

This rhythm is relatively rare in childhood especially outside hospital. As with adults, electrical cardioversion is the treatment of choice and should be performed without delay. The initial energy of the defibrillatory shock should be 2 J/kg, repeated once before increasing the energy to 4 J/kg for the third and subsequent defibrillation attempts. For older children the defibrillator electrodes are placed in the conventional positions on the chest wall, one below the right clavicle and the other in the left anterior axillary line below the cardiac apex. For infants it may be more appropriate to apply electrodes to the front and back of the chest. Paediatric electrodes should ideally be used in children below 10 kilograms but in larger children adult electrodes should be used provided the child's thorax is wide enough to permit electrode-to-skin contact over the entire electrode surface.

If ventricular fibrillation (or pulseless ventricular tachycardia) persists after the third defibrillatory shock, 1 minute of basic life support should be performed before a further batch of three shocks is given (all at the higher energy level). The cycle of defibrillatory shocks followed by 1 minute of basic life support must be repeated until defibrillation is achieved. Adrenaline is also recommended in the management of ventricular fibrillation and a dose of 10 μg per kilogram of body weight should be given after the first cycle of three shocks if the rhythm persists. A dose of 100 μg per kilogram is recommended after the second cycle of three shocks and between all subsequent cycles.

When ventricular fibrillation does occur in children, it is important to look for underlying causes – drug overdosage (particularly tricyclic antidepressants), hypothermia or electrolyte imbalance are particularly important. If attempts to reverse ventricular fibrillation outside hospital are unsuccessful and if the rhythm persists, consideration must be given to transferring the child to hospital, with basic life support in progress to maintain the cerebral and coronary circulation.

References and further reading

European Resuscitation Council (1998) Paediatric basic life support. *Resuscitation*, **37**:97–100.

European Resuscitation Council (1998) Paediatric advanced life support. *Resuscitation*, **37**:101–2.

International Liaison Committee on Resuscitation (1997) Paediatric life support: an advisory statement by the Paediatric Life Support Working Group of the International Liaison Committee on Resuscitation. *Resuscitation*, **34**:115–27.

Zideman DA (1997) Paediatric and neonatal life support. *British Journal of Anaesthesia*, **79**:178–187.

Zideman DA, Spearpoint K (1999) Resuscitation of infants and children. In *ABC of Resuscitation*, 4th edn (Colquhoun MC, Handley AJ, Evans TR, eds). BMJ Publishing Group, London.

Chapter 8

Resuscitation of the newly born

Introduction

In the 1960s approximately 25% of babies were delivered at home. During subsequent decades the proportion fell considerably with the centralization of maternity services within hospitals and, by 1994, only 2% of deliveries took place at home. In recent years there has been an increase in home births encouraged by the publication of the document 'Changing Childbirth' from the Department of Health (1993). Many general practitioners have little experience of managing labour and delivery in the home but are now more likely to be called to help, especially if unforeseen complications arise. It is therefore important that all GPs have a grasp of the fundamentals of resuscitation of the newly born; obviously members of the primary healthcare team who undertake intrapartum care will require special training and practice in these techniques.

The key to the safe practice of domiciliary obstetrics lies in careful patient selection. All babies suspected of being at increased risk at the time of delivery must be delivered in a unit with appropriate staff and equipment to provide resuscitation should it be necessary. About one-quarter of babies fall into this category of increased risk for one reason or another, and these account for around two-thirds of those requiring resuscitation. The remaining one-third are born after an uncomplicated labour with no apparent risk factors present. All staff attending apparently low risk births must therefore be prepared to provide adequate resuscitation until further expertise is available. To quote Changing Childbirth:

a woman giving birth at home or in a midwife/GP-led unit should feel confident that the midwife and doctor are able to provide help in the event of an acute emergency before transfer of mother and baby to a general hospital.

Preparations

Communication

Good communication between the midwife, primary healthcare team and the mother and her family is essential. With home deliveries the team will usually have had adequate time to establish a rapport with the mother, but this may not always be possible if unforeseen complications develop that require immediate intervention or the presence of further helpers. Lines of communication with the midwife and doctor need to be well defined before the onset of labour and the relevant phone numbers, pager numbers and the like must be known by all.

Equipment

The following resuscitation equipment is that recommended for home deliveries by the Royal College of Paediatrics and Child Health (1997):

- mobile phone or telephone within the home
- room heater and good light
- padded surface at table height
- gloves and warm towels
- self-inflating resuscitation bag, valve and facemasks, sizes 0, 00 and 000
- suction device and catheters
- resuscitation flow chart
- stop watch
- stethoscope
- oxygen cylinder with regulated flow rate of up to 10 l/min and an adjustable pressure release valve within the system
- syringes, needles and disposable sharps box
- torch
- checklist.

A dedicated resuscitation bag complete with an equipment inventory is ideal (Figure 8.1). Regular checks are essential to ensure that the equipment is functional and that used items are replaced.

The Resuscitation Council (UK) recommends that when birth takes place

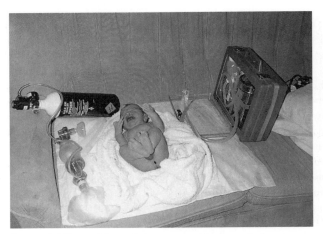

Figure 8.1 Home delivery: being prepared for resuscitation

in a non-designated delivery area the recommended minimum equipment should include a bag/valve/mask ventilation device of appropriate size for the newly born, a suction device with a selection of suitable catheters, warm dry towels and blankets, sterile equipment for cutting the umbilical cord and surgical gloves for the attendant. Whatever equipment is chosen it must be checked carefully and the attendant responsible for the care of the newborn baby must ensure that no item is missing and that all items are in working order. In most cases outside hospital this equipment will be carried by the midwives.

Personnel

Personnel trained in the basic skills of resuscitation at birth should be in attendance at every delivery and ideally at least one person should be responsible solely for the care of the infant. The Department of Health (1993) has recommended that ideally two trained professionals should be present (a midwife and doctor or two midwives), and stresses that one of these must be proficient at facemask resuscitation.

Thermal environment

A newborn baby tolerates a cold environment poorly and a wet newborn baby can cool rapidly after birth. Cold stress results in lower arterial oxygen saturations, increased oxygen consumption and impedes resuscitation. Wherever possible the baby should be delivered in a warm, draught-free room and dried as soon as practical after delivery. Wet linen should be removed immediately. Wrapping the infant in pre-warmed blankets will reduce heat loss and another strategy is to place the newly born baby on the mother's chest or abdomen to use her as a source of heat.

Universal precautions

All fluids from patients should be regarded as potentially infectious and personnel should wear appropriate protective clothing, including gloves and other barriers or shields as appropriate. Where a known risk of infection can be anticipated, delivery will normally be undertaken in hospital of course, but it is important to remember that between 15% and 35% of all home deliveries are unplanned.

Assessment at birth

Traditionally the APGAR scoring system has been widely used to indicate the need for resuscitation of newborn babies (Table 8.1).

Table 8.1 APGAR score chart

Score	0	1	2
Heart rate	Absent	<100 b.p.m.	100 b.p.m.
Respiratory effort	Absent	Irregular, slow	Regular, cry
Muscle tone	Limp	Some flexion in limbs	Well-flexed limbs
Reflex irritability	Nil	Grimace	Cough/cry
Colour	White	Blue	Pink

The need for resuscitation can usually be assessed more accurately by evaluating the heart rate, respiratory activity and colour of the baby than by the total APGAR score. The requirement to reassess the APGAR score after 1 minute may also lead to a delay in the initiation of resuscitation procedures. When required, resuscitation procedures should begin immediately after birth and continue until the vital signs are normal. In addition to the three cardinal signs mentioned above, the initial cry and

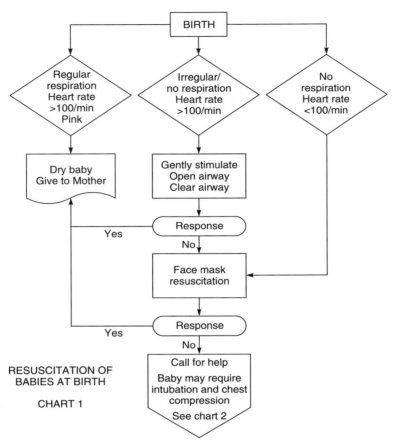

Note: If there is thick meconium and the baby is unresponsive, proceed immediately to chart 2

(a)

Figure 8.2 European Resuscitation Council Algorithm for Resuscitation of Babies at Birth – Charts 1 (a) and 2 (b) © ERC 1999 (from *European Resuscitation Council Guidelines for Resuscitation*, edited by L. Bossaert, 1998, Elsevier, Oxford by kind permission)

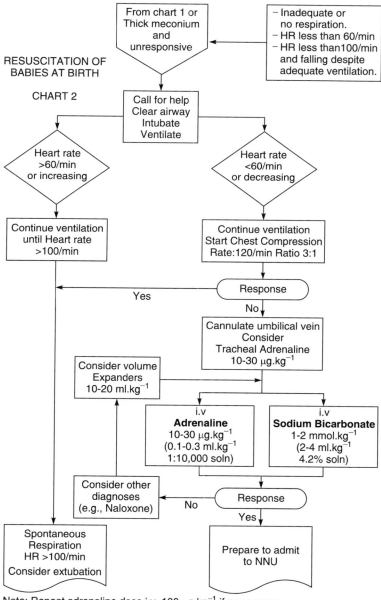

RESUSCITATION OF
BABIES AT BIRTH

CHART 2

From chart 1 or
Thick meconium
and
unresponsive

- Inadequate or
  no respiration.
- HR less than 60/min
- HR less than100/min
  and falling despite
  adequate ventilation.

Call for help
Clear airway
Intubate
Ventilate

Heart rate
>60/min
or increasing

Heart rate
<60/min
or decreasing

Continue ventilation
until Heart rate
>100/min

Continue ventilation
Start Chest Compression
Rate:120/min Ratio 3:1

Response

Yes

No

Cannulate umbilical vein
Consider
Tracheal Adrenaline
10-30 $\mu g.kg^{-1}$

Consider volume
Expanders
10-20 ml.kg^{-1}

i.v
Adrenaline
10-30 $\mu g.kg^{-1}$
(0.1-0.3 ml.kg^{-1}
1:10,000 soln)

i.v
Sodium Bicarbonate
1-2 mmol.kg^{-1}
(2-4 ml.kg^{-1}
4.2% soln)

Consider other
diagnoses
(e.g., Naloxone)

No

Response

Yes

Spontaneous
Respiration
HR >100/min

Consider extubation

Prepare to admit
to NNU

Note: Repeat adrenaline dose i.v. 100 $\mu g.kg^{-1}$ if no response

(b)

response to stimulation should be noted; simultaneous evaluation of all these signs (with action determined by the integrated findings) is more valuable than the evaluation of a single sign in isolation. The evaluation of the newborn infant is usually taught in following sequence.

Response to stimulation

Most newborn babies respond to the stimulation of the new environment in which they find themselves by moving the limbs, making strong respiratory efforts and giving a vigorous cry. If these responses are not present immediately after delivery, the child should be stimulated by drying with a towel, flicking the bottom of the feet, or rubbing the back. If these methods do not produce effective ventilation they should be abandoned because assisted ventilation is required. Slapping, shaking, spanking or holding the baby upside down by its feet are measures that are outmoded and potentially dangerous.

Respiration

After initial respiratory efforts (which may include a cry), the newly born baby should establish regular respiration. The rate, depth and symmetry of respiration should be noted and any abnormal movements, such as gasping or grunting, are abnormal and may require intervention.

Heart rate

The heart rate should be determined by listening to the heart through a stethoscope placed on the precordium. Feeling for the pulsation of the umbilical artery at the base of the cord is an alternative method. The heart rate should be greater than 100 beats per minute; increases or decreases in rate may imply improvement or deterioration in the infant's condition respectively and should be observed carefully.

Colour

The normal infant will maintain a pink coloration while breathing room air. The presence of central cyanosis should be determined by examining the mucous membranes, for example in the mouth. Its presence signifies failure of oxygenation of blood within the heart and pulmonary circulation. Peripheral cyanosis is common and by itself is not an adverse finding.

Classification according to initial assessment

Following the initial assessment babies can be placed in one of four categories.

1. Fit and healthy baby

This baby has vigorous effective respiratory efforts and is pink with a heart rate of over 100 beats per minute. This will be the anticipated outcome in all planned deliveries outside hospital and no intervention beyond drying the baby and wrapping it in a warm towel is required before handing it to the mother.

2. Inadequate breathing

This baby will show inadequate respiratory efforts or may be centrally cyanosed but will usually have a heart rate of more than 100 beats per minute. Tactile stimulation, with or without oxygen delivered by a facemask, will often correct the situation but, if these measures are unsuccessful, basic life support will be required.

3. Inadequate breathing or apnoeic

Pale or white (because of poor cardiac output and peripheral vasoconstriction). The heart rate is usually less than 100 beats per minute. This is a nightmare scenario to confront those caring for a mother and baby at home or in the GP Obstetric Unit. Expert help must obviously be summoned, however possible, while basic life support is instigated. Immediate intubation with positive pressure ventilation is usually highly desirable if at all possible with the resources available.

4. Pale or white but no detectable heart rate

If it were possible to imagine a worse scenario than (3) above, this is it. Immediate ventilation, chest compression and full advanced life support procedures, including the use of drugs, is required while help is summoned. The ability to provide this will obviously depend on the equipment and personnel available.

Basic life support

This should be started if the baby has not cried after 30 seconds or established regular respiration by 1 minute after birth. If a heart rate below 100 beats per minute can be accurately documented at this time, then this is an additional indication. As with adults, basic life support follows the usual ABC sequence.

a) Airway

The baby should be placed on his or her back with the neck in a neutral or slightly extended position. Be careful not to overextend the neck because this may produce airway obstruction by stretching the airways in the neck. If respiratory efforts are present but not producing adequate ventilation, the airway is obstructed and efforts must be made to clear it. The usual cause of airway obstruction will be amniotic fluid and perhaps meconium; gentle suction to the upper airway will usually resolve matters. Aggressive suction should be avoided as this may cause laryngeal spasm and vagally-induced bradycardia. It should not be necessary to insert a suction catheter more than 5 cm from the lips of the baby.

b) Breathing

Assisted ventilation should be provided if the infant is apnoeic, gasping or if the heart rate remains under 100 beats per minute despite tactile stimulation. The best method for assisting ventilation is with a bag/valve/mask device, but when equipment is not available, mouth-to-mouth/nose ventilation is effective. Consensus continues to support initial attempts at ventilation by both the mouth and nose and a well-fitting facemask, which covers both forming an adequate seal, is preferable to produce effective inflation of the lungs. A round mask with a soft continuous cuff which seals against the face is the recommended device to achieve this. Ventilation can be provided either by a self-inflating bag (Figure 8.3), or by feeding air or oxygen into one arm of a T-piece attached to the facemask. With the latter system the baby's lungs are inflated by occluding the open arm of the T-piece. Whichever method is used, a safety device to limit inflation pressure to 20–30 cm water must be incorporated. Ventilation should be provided at a rate of 30 per minute allowing one second for both inspiration and expiration. The effectiveness of ventilation is assessed by observing movements of the chest wall and improvement in the baby's colour and heart rate.

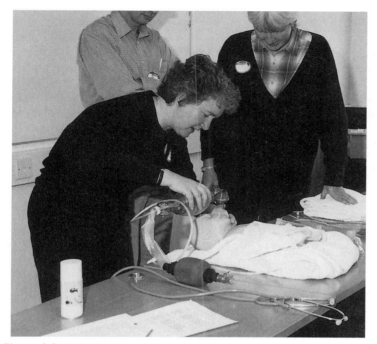

Figure 8.3 Ventilation using a self-inflating bag

It is often recommended that the technique is modified for the first few breaths so that the inspiratory phase is prolonged for 1–2 seconds to ensure full lung expansion.

If the heart rate is more than 100 beats per minute ventilation should be continued until spontaneous respiration is established. If the baby does not respond to facemask resuscitation, it is often recommended that tracheal intubation is performed, but this may not be possible outside hospital. If the heart rate is falling, chest compressions should be initiated while further help is summoned or arrangements are made to transfer the baby to hospital.

c) Circulation

The circulation is assessed by evaluating the heart rate and colour of the baby. The heart rate is monitored by auscultation of the heart with a stethoscope on the precordium or by palpation of the umbilical artery at the base of the cord. A rate of greater than 100 beats per minute indicates the need to continue monitoring and assessment, while if it is less than 100 beats per minute and decreasing, positive pressure ventilation should be carried out. Chest compressions should be started if asystole is present or if the heart rate is less than 60 beats per minute despite adequate assisted ventilation for 30 seconds. The establishment of adequate ventilation will restore the circulation in the great majority of newborn infants, and because chest compressions may diminish the effectiveness of ventilation they should not be initiated until effective ventilation has been established.

Compressions should be applied to the lower third of the sternum and should be delivered with a force sufficient to compress the anteroposterior diameter of the chest by approximately one-third. Two techniques are in general use. In the first, the thumbs of the rescuer are placed on the sternum superimposed or adjacent to each other depending on the size of the baby, with fingers surrounding the thorax (Figure 8.4). With the second technique the index and middle finger of one hand are used to compress the lower sternum (Figure 8.5). This technique is thought to be less effective but does leave the remaining hand free for other tasks. The compressions should be smooth, not jerky, and each should last about 50% of the compression/relaxation cycle. The thumbs or fingers should not be lifted off the sternum during the relaxation phase but the chest wall should be allowed to return to its resting position between each compression. A ratio of three compressions to one ventilation is recommended so that 90 compressions and 30 breaths are achieved every minute. The presence of a spontaneous pulse should be checked after 1 minute and periodically thereafter and compressions continued until the natural heart rate is greater than 60.

Meconium aspiration

Light staining of the amniotic fluid is not necessarily an indication for any intervention if the baby is well. If lumpy meconium is passed per vagina, the nose should be gently aspirated as soon as the head is delivered. If the baby is subsequently well no further action may be required. If the baby is not vigorous, direct laryngoscopy should be carried out and if this shows meconium in the pharynx and trachea the baby should ideally be intubated and suction applied to the tracheal tube while it is removed. Provided the baby's heart rate remains above 60 beats per minute this procedure can be

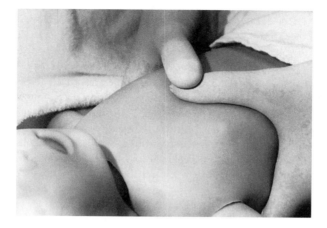

Figure 8.4 Chest compressions – the two-thumb technique

repeated until no further meconium is recovered. Tracheal suction of a vigorous infant with meconium-stained fluid is not likely to be helpful and may cause later problems.

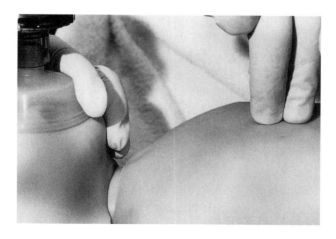

Figure 8.5 Chest compressions – two-finger technique

Advanced life support

More advanced life support techniques, including advanced airway procedures, intravenous access and the use of drugs, is beyond the scope of this book. GPs who undertake regular intrapartum care (especially in units where an anaesthetist or paediatrician are not immediately available) will require knowledge of these procedures. The further reading section at the end of the chapter contains appropriate references and the Neonatal Life Support course administered by the Resuscitation Council (UK) provides a standardized course where the important techniques of neonatal resuscitation can be learned and practised.

Transfer of mother and baby

The Department of Health (1993) considers it essential that 'clear guidelines' for the management of neonatal emergencies occurring in the community are drawn up. It is intended that these should cover the immediate care and transfer of newly born infants who require further treatment or assessment in the neonatal unit. Details of such guidelines will depend much on local circumstances and resources and should be formulated with the agreement of all parties involved in the care of the mother and child, both in the community and after their subsequent transfer to hospital.

Communication with the parents

The team caring for the newborn baby should inform the parents of the baby's progress, the procedures being undertaken (and why they are required). It is important to be as frank and honest as circumstances permit, but it will not usually be possible in the circumstances under discussion to give accurate prognostic information.

References and further reading

Confidential Enquiry into Stillbirths and Deaths in Infancy (1998) *5th Annual Report*. Maternal and Child Health Research Consortium, London.

Davies J, Hey E, Reid W *et al.* (1996) Prospective regional study of planned home birth. *Br Med J,* **313**:1302–5.

Department of Health (1993) *Changing Childbirth.* HMSO, London.

European Resuscitation Council (1998) *The 1998 European Resuscitation Council Guidelines for the Resuscitation of Babies at Birth in European Resuscitation Council Guidelines for Resuscitation* (Bossaert L, ed.). pp 101–16. Elsevier, Oxford.

Hamilton P (1999) Care of new born in the delivery room. In *The ABC of Labour Care* (Chamberlain G, ed.). BMJ Publishing Group, London.

Kattwinkel J, Niermeyers, Nadkarni *et al.* (1999) Resuscitation of a newly born infant: advisory statement from Paediatric Working Group of the International Liaison Committee on Resuscitation. *Resuscitation,* **40**:71–88.

Millner AD (1999) Resuscitation at birth. In *The ABC of Resuscitation,* 4th edn (Colquhoun MC, Handley AJ, Evans TR, eds). BMJ Publishing Group, London.

North West Thames Health Authority (1994) *North West Thames Annual Maternity Figures (1992 & 1993).* London Office for National Statistics, HMSO, London.

Chapter 9

Ethical and practical issues applied to resuscitation outside hospital

Ethical issues related to resuscitation

The application of modern knowledge and technology has made it possible to resuscitate patients who would otherwise not survive and many long-term survivors of cardiac arrest or other life-threatening illness testify to the value and effectiveness of modern resuscitation techniques.

The aims of modern resuscitation medicine are the same as the goals of most medical interventions – the preservation of life and the maintenance of health. Among the victims of cardiac arrest, however, many will not survive and these patients (and perhaps their relatives) are needlessly exposed to an unnecessary and undignified procedure producing no benefit. Unfortunately, there is no way at present to predict accurately which patients will survive and, by default, resuscitation attempts are made in most patients who collapse. The reported success rates for out of hospital resuscitation vary between 2 and 20%, emphasizing the fact that resuscitation is inappropriate for many patients. In those patients in whom the circulation is initially restored around 30% die later in hospital and resuscitation can be viewed as an extension of the process of dying imposing considerable suffering for the patient and their relatives. A further proportion of survivors suffer neurological disabilities or other adverse consequences.

In an ideal world resuscitation would only be started in those patients likely to survive. Cardiac arrest occurring outside hospital is usually a sudden event occurring in people who are previously well; in an emergency situation immediate action is required. In many cases the likelihood of success, the previous health and quality of life of the patient and indeed, the wishes of the patient and their relatives are unknown.

The obligation on those who might attempt the resuscitation of these patients (or who plan the medical systems responsible) is to decide, in advance, the best way to recognize those patients who have no chance of survival (where the resuscitation attempt is futile), and where resuscitation should be withheld for other reasons. No comprehensive formal guidelines exist to address these issues although consensus among experts is beginning to emerge.

The complexity of the problem is confounded by a patient's right to make their own decisions about treatment – patient autonomy. Furthermore, the right to accept or reject medical care continues after the patient has lost the capacity to make this decision. Advanced directives or living wills would direct treatment in this situation but, in practice, the patients previous wishes are often unknown. A refusal to undergo treatment made by a mentally competent patient who has been adequately informed is legally binding on doctors. Members of the primary health care team are occasionally asked by patients, particularly the elderly, about being spared unpleasant, invasive procedures, when there is little likelihood of survival. This opportunity might also be used to explore feelings about resuscitation in the event of sudden collapse. Studies have shown that elderly patients are often less enthusiastic about resuscitation procedures when better informed about the consequences and likely chances of success.

In the community, resuscitation may be attempted inappropriately by doctors, other members of the health care team or by the ambulance service who do not know the full circumstances of the patient. In some cases the ambulance service are bound to follow protocols or standing orders.

There is much that can be done to avoid this situation and, in many cases, inappropriate resuscitation attempts can be prevented by the application of a Do-Not-Resuscitate (DNR) decision.

Do-Not-Resuscitate (DNR) decisions

In the authors' experience problems arise when the staff of nursing homes, rest homes or community hospitals – with the best of intentions – initiate inappropriate resuscitation attempts. The situation will be confounded if the ambulance service is summoned to help. The latter will often be duty bound to continue a resuscitation attempt until orders to the contrary have been issued and this may mean summoning a doctor to attend or transporting a patient to the local A & E department with resuscitation in progress.

A similar situation arises when well-meaning relatives of a patient who is terminally ill summon the ambulance service when a patient actually dies, perhaps because of a perception that agonal respirations or gasps indicate that the patient is distressed; a conscious decision not to resuscitate such a patient can prevent this unfortunate situation. Considerable discussion with the patient and their relatives will be required and adequate time must be allowed to answer questions from relatives and carers. This is particularly the case when lay personnel are involved.

Considerable advances in the establishment of formal do-not-resuscitate polices have taken place in hospital practice in recent years, and guidelines have been formulated by the British Medical Association, the Royal College of Nursing and the Resuscitation Council (UK). The principles contained in these guidelines are equally applicable in nursing homes, rest homes, community hospitals or other environments where patients may collapse or die and resuscitation be attempted inappropriately. It is quite appropriate to consider a do-not-resuscitate decision in the community in the following circumstances:

- Where a patient's illness means that resuscitation is unlikely to be successful.
- Where successful resuscitation is likely to be followed by length or quality of life that would not be in the best interests of the patient to sustain.
- Where a mentally competent patient has indicated that resuscitation is not wanted. This wish may be stated during the course of an illness or may have being made previously in an advance directive or living will (Figure 9.1).

Where a DNR decision is made because of the absence of any likely benefit, discussion with the patient or their relatives should take place to ensure that the reasons for the decision have been fully understood and accepted. Where the decision is based on the likely quality of life in the event of successful resuscitation, the views of the patient, family, or close friends should be sought to ascertain what would be in the patient's best interests. Such discussions involve complex issues in a highly sensitive area and should be undertaken by experienced staff who know the patient and their circumstances. It must be stressed that a DNR decision applies only to resuscitation procedures and that all other treatment and nursing procedures will be unaffected by any such decision.

The overall responsibility for a DNR decision in the community will usually rest with the general practitioner in charge of the patient's care. He or she will usually be best placed to consider the most important aspects of the patient's condition and take into account the views of the patient,

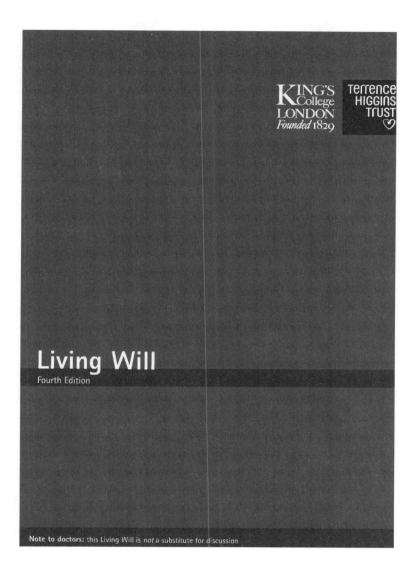

Figure 9.1 A living will

others members of the primary health care team and relatives or close friends. The importance of team work in this situation cannot be over emphasized.

Accurate record keeping and communication are the key to the successful formulation and application of any DNR decision. The patient's notes should record the decision accurately and the reason for this; as in hospital practice this should be signed and dated by the general practitioner responsible. Where appropriate, nursing records should also make it clear that the decision exists and a management structure should be in place to ensure that all who care for the patient are aware of the decision. This poses considerable practical problems considering the number of agencies often involved and the way that terminal care is organized in the community.

Futile resuscitation

It is possible to identify some situations where there is absolutely no chance of survival and where resuscitation would be both futile and also distressing for relatives, friends and the health care personnel involved. Guidance to help in this situation has been provided by the Joint Royal Colleges' Ambulance Service Liaison Committee in response to requests from ambulance services NHS trusts. A key point is that there is a great difference between the recognition that someone has died and the formal certification of death which can only be undertaken (in the UK) by a registered medical practitioner. While recognizing that it is essential that death is not erroneously diagnosed and a potential survivor denied treatment, simple guidelines have been formulated to help identify conditions unequivocally associated with death. In other cases an ECG will assist the diagnosis.

Conditions unequivocally associated with death

- Decapitation
- Massive cranial and cerebral destruction
- Hemi-corporectomy (or similar massive injury)
- Decomposition
- Incineration
- Rigor mortis
- Fetal maceration.

In this group of patients death may be recognized by the finding of cardiac arrest.

Conditions requiring ECG evidence of asystole

- A submersion for more than 3 hours in adults over 18 years of age (with or without hypothermia).
- Continuous asystole despite cardiopulmonary resuscitation for more than 20 minutes in normothermic patients.
- Patients who have received no resuscitation for at least 15 minutes after collapse and who have no pulse or respiratory effort on the arrival of the ambulance personnel.

In all these categories it is essential that the timings are accurate. In all cases the ECG must be recorded accurately, and must be free from artefact and unequivocally demonstrate asystole. There must be no history of sedative, hypnotic, opiate or anaesthetic drug administration in the preceding 24 hours. These guidelines have been adopted by several ambulance services and used successfully; the principles contained therein apply equally to other health care providers in the community.

When to stop resuscitation

If resuscitation does not result in the return of a spontaneous circulation, there are two basic options open to those treating a patient in the out of hospital environment. The first is to terminate the resuscitation attempt at the scene, while the second is to transport the patient to hospital with on-going basic life support in progress. There are no strict rules, but both the American Heart Association (AHA) and the European Resuscitation Council (ERC) have published general guidance to justify terminating a resuscitation attempt. The ERC guidelines are more specific but neither organization defines the exact time when resuscitation should be abandoned. Both provide a framework within which to exercise individual judgement. The ERC guidelines also emphasize conditions that justify prolonged resuscitation attempts; these include drug intoxication, hypothermia and treatment for potentially correctable conditions, for example tension pneumothorax. Study of the application of these guidelines has shown that hospital-based cardiac arrest teams used additional criteria to decide when to cease resuscitation efforts and that the ERC and AHA criteria were not sufficiently comprehensive to cover all the situations encountered.

The ERC guidelines consider the following factors:

- The environment and access to emergency medical services. A cardiac arrest occurring in a remote area where access to emergency medical services is limited or delayed is associated with a poor outcome unless a spontaneous circulation can be restored with basic life support.
- The interval between the onset of cardiopulmonary arrest and the application of basic life support. If this interval is more than 5 minutes (assessed accurately), the prognosis is poor and there is a substantial risk of neurological deficit. Evidence from the Scottish Ambulance Service has suggested that resuscitation attempts should be abandoned in patients in cardiac arrest if the time from the collapse to the arrival of the ambulance exceeds 15 minutes if no attempts at CPR have been made and the ECG shows an unshockable rhythm. This recommendation was supported by a study of 414 patients who had not received CPR in 15 or more minutes prior to the arrival of the ambulance and has been incorporated into formal guidelines for ambulance personnel.
- Interval between starting basic life support and the institution of advanced life support measures. Survival from cardiac arrest is rare if defibrillation or drug treatment is not available within 20 minutes (provided basic life support has been present for this time). Each case must be judged on an individual basis taking into account evidence of cardiac death, cerebral damage, the ultimate prognosis and age of the patient. Hypothermia (particularly in children) is a favourable sign and prolonged resuscitation attempts are justified.
- Evidence of cardiac death. In one large study of nearly 1500 patients there were no survivors in those with asystole persisting longer than 20 minutes. Patients in asystole who are unresponsive to adrenaline and fluid replacement are unlikely to survive and the ERC guidelines recommend that resuscitation should be abandoned after 15 minutes. Obviously patients with persistent ventricular fibrillation should be actively treated until a spontaneous circulation is established or asystole or electromechanical dissociation supervene.
- Evidence of cerebral damage. Persistently fixed and dilated pupils (when not related to previous drug administration) are an indication of serious cerebral damage and, in the absence of other possible causes, it

is recommended that serious consideration is given to abandoning the resuscitation attempt.

- Potential prognosis and underlying disease. Where resuscitation has been started in patients with a very poor ultimate prognosis or with end-stage disease the attempt should be abandoned early on. Prolonged resuscitation attempts in this group of patients are rarely successful and there is a high incidence of cerebral damage in this group.
- Age in itself has a relatively minor impact on outcome. The latter is more affected by the underlying disease process causing the arrest. This is thought to be the explanation for lower survival rates in patients in their 70s and 80s. The ERC recommendations are for earlier curtailment of resuscitative efforts in the elderly. Children, however, are more tolerant of hypoxia and prolonged resuscitation attempts are justified.
- Temperature: hypothermia provides protection against the effects of hypoxia, particularly in the brain, and resuscitation should be continued for longer in these patients. It is recommended that resuscitation should be continued in hypothermic patients while re-warming is carried out. This group of patients more than any other have the most to gain from the continuation of basic life support during transport to hospital where active re-warming can be performed.
- Drug intake before cardiac arrest − sedative, hypnotic or narcotic drugs are said to provide a degree of cerebral protection if taken before the arrest and again prolonged resuscitation attempts are often justified.
- Remedial factors. Where the possibility of a potentially remedial condition exists, resuscitation should continue. Tension pneumothorax and cardiac tamponade are two examples of such conditions where intervention may prove life saving. The outcome following cardiac arrest secondary to trauma is notoriously poor and the availability of skilled surgery and rapid transfusion facilities need to be taken into account if the resuscitation attempt is prolonged.

Conclusion

The ethical principles that apply to out of hospital resuscitation are not greatly different from those applied to the treatment of other conditions or resuscitation in other circumstances. They are, however, applied in a special situation characterized by limited time, a lack of accurate diagnostic information, limited therapeutic possibilities and a severely curtailed relationship between the patient and health care providers. The same principle of providing treatment to preserve life, restore health and the relief of suffering remains, as does the principle of avoiding procedures with potential adverse consequences. The principles of patient autonomy and consent remain even though the patient may be unable to communicate their wishes at the time.

References and further reading

Baskett PJF (1993) Ethics in cardiopulmonary resuscitation. *Resuscitation,* **25**:1–8.
Baskett, PJF (1999) The ethics of resuscitation. In *The ABC of Resuscitation,* 4th edn (Colquhoun MC, Handley AJ, Evans TR, eds). BMJ Publishing Group, London.
Bossaert L (1994) *The Ethics of Resuscitation in Clinical Practice, a Statement on Behalf of the European Resuscitation Council,* pp. 210–17. Elsevier Science.
European Resuscitation Council (1998) Ethical principles in out of hospital cardiopulmonary resuscitation. In *European Resuscitation Council Guidelines for Resuscitation* (Bossaert L, ed.), pp. 206–9. Elsevier Science.
Holmberg S, Ekstro ML (1992) Ethics and practicalities of resuscitation, a statement for the Advanced Life Support Working Party of the European Resuscitation Council. *Resuscitation,* **24**:239–44.

Chapter 10

Learning resuscitation techniques

The methods used to teach resuscitation skills have been the subject of much investigation in recent years. Considerable effort has been devoted by teachers and educationists into the best method of teaching resuscitation techniques so that the skills involved are easily acquired and retained. There is an extensive literature largely derived from hospital-based studies and well researched data are available on:

- The optimal methods of teaching and class design.
- The adaptation of teaching techniques to adult learners.
- Skill acquisition in various class settings.
- Skill retention after initial instruction.

Although very few specific studies have been carried out in general practice, the knowledge we have is equally applicable outside hospital. Several studies performed in the 1980s demonstrated the inability of trained nurses and doctors to perform cardiopulmonary resuscitation adequately, and this led to a wide-ranging review of training methods within the National Health Service. A key development was the Royal College of Physician's report 'Resuscitation from Cardiopulmonary Arrest: Training and Organisation (1987)', which revolutionized resuscitation training within hospitals, largely through the establishment of the Resuscitation Training Officers. Further studies, unfortunately, continued to show poor skill retention by health care professionals (as well as the public) and there is unfortunately, no consensus on the best way to overcome the problem nor on how often refresher courses are required. Poor skill retention has been demonstrated as little as 2 weeks after attending a training class and if subjects are formally evaluated 1 year after training, their skill level is often similar to that before training took place. The degree of skill retention does not necessarily correlate with the thoroughness of initial training and when candidates have been assessed as being fully competent at the end of a training session, skill decay still occurs rapidly. It has been shown, rather worryingly, that both doctors and nurses cannot accurately predict their level of knowledge or skill at performing basic resuscitation techniques before formal evaluation. In several groups of health care professionals the confidence in their ability to perform resuscitation has been shown to correlate very poorly with competence when assessed objectively.

Simplification of the course content, repetition of the teaching and manikin practice are the only measures shown to maximize recall. There is no evidence that experience acquired at real cardiac arrests improves theoretical knowledge or skills — only repeated refresher training courses have been shown to facilitate the retention of the psychomotor skills involved.

Levels of training

Resuscitation training may conveniently be catagorized into different levels of attainment.

Basic life support (Chapter 2)

All health care staff who are in contact with patients should be trained to perform basic life support and this will mean that practically the whole primary health care team should be trained. Regular refresher courses and manikin practice are required to maintain skill levels.

Basic life support with airway adjunct

Airway adjuncts is the term used to describe the protective facemasks and shields. Their use should be learned (and practised on manikins) by all health care workers. Increasingly first aiders and the general public request training in the use of these aids.

Basic life support with airway adjuncts plus defibrillation

The advent of the automated external defibrillator (AED) has bought this level of skill attainment within the capability of a very wide range of health care professionals. Increasingly nurses on general wards defibrillate patients using an AED before the arrival of the cardiac arrest team. The sooner the defibrillatory shock is applied, the greater the chance of success and this has been reflected in beneficial results reported following the introduction of policies that enable early defibrillation. With the simplicity of use provided by modern first responder defibrillators, practically all members of the primary health care team would be capable of reaching this level of skill attainment. Defibrillation is the procedure that saves the most lives and the more people who can do it the better, so that the delay in administering the shock can be minimized.

Advanced life support (Chapter 3)

Outside hospital advanced life support techniques are taught to paramedics and many GPs also acquire these skills. Formal training (and refresher courses) will certainly be needed by doctors who work with the ambulance service as part of an immediate care scheme.

Learning resuscitation

The practice of resuscitation requires skills that are essentially practical and practical training is necessary to acquire them. Sophisticated training manikins and other teaching aids greatly assist this process, but it is simplification of the course content, repetition of the theory and repeated practice that is the key to success. This is not easy to arrange in general practice with the many competing demands on limited time for postgraduate education, but once the skills have been acquired refresher practice and updating are not particularly time consuming nor arduous. The main problem is presented by limited access to training manikins and the services of a Resuscitation Training Officer, but the situation has improved greatly in recent years.

The teaching and acquisition of resuscitation skills has been more intensively studied than practically any other area of medical education. Certain key factors in the success of this aim are established. In the first place it is essential that the classes include not only theoretical instruction but also practice on manikins of the techniques being taught. The greater the time devoted to manikin practice, the better the skills will be learned and remembered. Most resuscitation courses are designed for adults who are usually well motivated to learn once they have decided to acquire the skills; this requires motivation which is increased if the purpose of the teaching is clear and relevant to the individual's needs (Figure 10.1). Adults

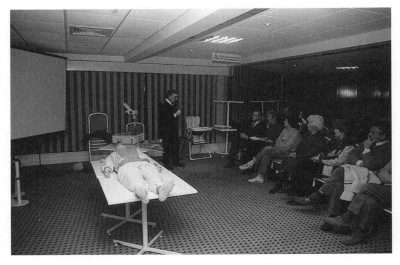

Figure 10.1 Basic life support training (HeartStart)

usually learn best when treated as adults and when the wealth of personal experience that they bring to the class is recognized. It is important that 'the self' is not threatened – for example by ridicule (however light hearted) in the event of poor performance.

Active participation in the class with self-evaluation and feedback about performance is important in the teaching of psychomotor skills (Figure 10.2). Feedback is traditionally categorized as intrinsic or extrinsic – intrinsic feedback is the sensory information that students receive while performing a task, while extrinsic feedback is objective information about performance. Sophisticated training manikins provide detailed information about performance and have the advantage over the use of checklists or video recordings as the data may be made confidential with the results available only to the learners.

Teaching in small groups (with 4–6 trainees per manikin) should allow sufficient time to practise skills and receive feedback about performance. One method of providing feedback is to ask members of the class to provide a critique on a student's performance on a manikin.

Simulated cardiac arrest scenarios are a further method of teaching resuscitation skills and help develop team work and place the subject in context. Such scenarios may logically follow on from the teaching and practice of individual skills like basic life support or defibrillation. A more

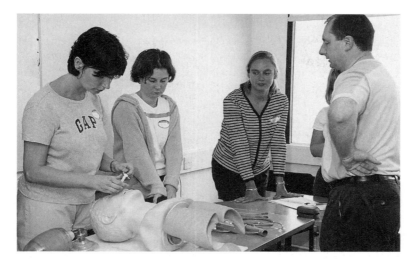

Figure 10.2 Learning a skill

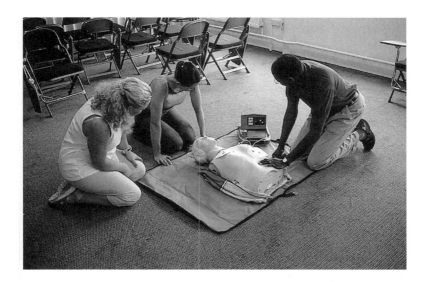

Figure 10.3 AED training

immediate perspective will result if the scenario takes place in the work place, for example with the manikin representing the collapsed patient being placed in the waiting room. Such scenarios help bridge the gap between theory and practice and help improve communication and decision making. They have also been shown to reduce anxiety levels.

Resuscitation courses

Resuscitation Council (UK) Advanced Life Support course

The ALS course is designed to teach the theory and practical skills required to manage cardiopulmonary arrest in adults from the time when the arrest seems imminent until the patient is transferred to an intensive care department or dies. It is run over a minimum of 2 days and consists of lectures, practical stations and assessments. A manual is sent 1 month before the course and the candidate is advised to study this thoroughly before completing a pre-course multiple choice paper. Competence in basic life support is expected and is tested after a brief demonstration on the first day of the course. Although the course is primarily designed for those who practise resuscitation in hospital, the skills acquired are equally applicable outside hospital and many GPs have attended ALS courses. For further information contact the ALS Course Coordinator at the Resuscitation Council (UK).

Resuscitation Council (UK) NLS course

The Resuscitation Council (UK) approved Neonatal Life Support course (NLS) is a recently introduced course and is run by a few centres at present. It is a 1- or 2-day practically orientated course covering the important aspects of neonatal resuscitation. Further information is available from the Resuscitation Council (UK).

Resuscitation Council (UK) Paediatric Advanced Life Support (PALS) course

The main emphasis of the 2-day PALS course is the recognition of the child in incipient or established respiratory or circulatory failure and the development of the knowledge and skills required to intervene to prevent further deterioration towards arrest.

Further information is available from the Resuscitation Council (UK). Very similar material is covered in the APLS (Advanced Paediatric Life Support course) administered by the Advanced Life Support Group (ALSG) in Manchester.

Paediatric Life Support course

The PLS course is similar to the PALS course, but is run over only 1 day. It is overseen by the ALSG in Manchester.

BASICS courses

The British Association of Immediate Care Schemes (BASICS) offer a range of courses for those interested in immediate medical care, especially in the pre-hospital arena. The organization was founded by general practitioners, and GPs maintain an active role in the running of the organization. Courses currently available include The Immediate Care course (ICC) – a detailed 5-day residential course where the pre-hospital management of both trauma and medical emergencies is taught. The Pre-hospital Emergency Care course (PHEC) is a shorter course and necessarily less detailed. Refresher courses and driving courses are also available. Further information is available from BASICS.

The British Red Cross

The British Red Cross runs several first aid courses including:

- HSE First Aid at Work
- HSE First Aid at Work re-qualification course
- Appointed Person First Aid course
- Basic First Aid course
- First Aid for Child Carers
- Emergency First Aid
- Save a Life course
- AED course.

For further information contact the British Red Cross Society.

The Basic First Aid course (or the equivalent run by the other voluntary aid bodies or the Royal Life Saving Society) provides instruction in basic life support as well as the principles of first aid that are ideally suited to the non-clinical members of the practice team, particularly receptionists or secretarial staff who may have to deal with an emergency when no doctors or nurses are available. Instruction in the use of automated defibrillators is also available through these organizations which should be contacted directly.

St John Ambulance

The St John Ambulance runs a number of first aid courses including:

- HSE First Aid at Work
- HSE First Aid at Work re-qualification course
- Appointed Person First Aid course
- First Aid for Child Carers
- AED course.

St Andrew's Ambulance Association

The St Andrew's Ambulance Association runs several first aid courses including:

- HSE First Aid at Work
- HSE First Aid at Work re-qualification course
- Appointed Person First Aid course
- First Aid for Child Carers
- Emergency First Aid
- AED course.

The Royal Life Saving Society UK

The Royal Life Saving Society is the principal provider of lifeguard training in the UK. The basic skills of the lifeguard – prevention, rescue and resuscitation – are taught to over 250 000 young people and adults every year. Training at both basic and advanced levels is available. Courses offered include:

- Life Support
- Lifeguard Training
- Life Saving
- AED courses.

Further information is available from the head office of the Royal Life Saving Society.

The British Heart Foundation

In recent years the British Heart Foundation, through its Heartstart UK initiative, has played a key role in the establishment of a nationwide network of organizations providing instruction in emergency life support skills. The classes occupy a single session and last for between 2 and 3 hours. At the time of writing there are 500 affiliated schemes and many offer training for GPs and their reception staff. In one study of GPs' basic life support skills, the practice that had held a refresher course run by a local Heartstart group performed very much better than the other GPs assessed. The Foundation's role is one of facilitation and coordination and in a relatively short time an impressive network of expertise has been built up, with GPs playing a key role in the formation and running of many schemes in their practice areas.

Useful addresses

Resuscitation Council UK
5th Floor Tavistock House North
Tavistock Square
London WC1H 9JR
Tel: 020 7388 4678

British Heart Foundation
14 Fitzhardinge Street
London W1H 4DH
Tel: 020 935 0185

British Red Cross Society
9 Grosvenor Crescent
London SW1X 7EJ
Tel: 020 7235 5454

St John Ambulance
1 Grosvenor Crescent
London SW1X 7EF
Tel: 020 7235 5231

St Andrew's Ambulance Association
St Andrew's House
48 Milton Street
Glasgow G4 0HR
Tel: 0141 332 4031

The Royal Life Saving Society UK
River House
High Street
Broom
Warwickshire B50 4HN
Tel: 01789 773994

BASICS
7 Blackhorse Lane
Ipswich
Suffolk IP1 2EF
Tel: 01473 218407

Advanced Life Support Group (ALSG)
2nd Floor, The Dock Office
Trafford Road
Salford Quays
Manchester M5 2XB
Tel: 0161 877 1999

Training manikins and other resuscitation equipment are available from a
number of companies including:
Laerdal Medical
Laerdal House
Goodmeade Road
Orpington
Kent BR6 OHX
Tel: 0168 9876634

Medtronic Physio-Control
Leamington Court
Andover House
Newfound
Basingstoke
Hampshire RG23 7HE
Tel: 01256 782727

Timesco of London
Timesco House
1 Knights Road
London E16 2AT
Tel: 020 7511 1234

References and further reading

Colquhoun M, Simons R (1999) Training manikins in teaching resuscitation. In *ABC of Resuscitation*, 4th edn (Colquhoun MC, Handley AJ, Evans TR, eds). BMJ Publishing Group, London.

Kaye W, Menziney M, Rallis S *et al.* (1989) Educational aspects: resuscitation training and evaluation clinics. In *Critical Care Medicine*. Churchill Livingstone, Edinburgh.

Resuscitation Council UK (1998) *Resuscitation for the Citizen*, 5th edn. Resuscitation Council, London.

Wynne G, Gwinnutt C, Bingham R *et al.* (1999) Teaching resuscitation. In *ABC of Resuscitation*, 4th edn (Colquhoun MC, Handley AJ, Evans TR, eds). BMJ Publishing Group, London.

Index

ABC mnemonic for basic life support, 11
Abdominal thrusts, 89–90
Adenosine, 73
Adrenaline, 37–9, 40
  anaphylaxis, 78–80
  bradycardia, 70
  children, 96, 98–9
  endobronchial, 37
  non-VF/VT rhythms, 35
  ventricular fibrillation/tachycardia, 32, 98–9
Advance directives, 116
Advanced life support, 7–8
  children and infants, 90–9
  drug administration, 36–40, 94–6
  hypothermia, 60
  impact of time to implementation, 120
  non-VF/VT rhythms, 34–6
  training, 8, 125, 128
  trauma cases, 66–8
  universal algorithm, 28–30
  ventricular fibrillation, 30–4
Age and outcome of resuscitation, 121
Airway management
  artificial airways, 45–51
  assessment, 11–13, 42–3
  basic life support in adults, 11–15
  children and infants, 84–6, 90–3
  newborn babies, 108
  manoeuvres to open and clear airway, 43–4
  suction, 45
  see also Ventilation
Alkalizing agents, 40, 98
Ambulance service
  advisory defibrillators, 26
  response to chest pain, 4

Amiodarone, 39–40
Anaphylaxis, 75–8
  treatment algorithms, 76–81
Antiarrhythmic drugs, 32, 39–40
Antihistamines, 80
APGAR scoring, 103
Asthma and cardiopulmonary arrest, 64–5
Asystole, 5–6
  adults, 34–6
  children, 96–8
  conditions requiring ECG evidence, 119
  impact of duration, 120
Atropine
  asystole, 35–6
  bradycardia, 39, 40, 70
  endobronchial, 37

Back blows, 18–19, 89
Barrier devices for ventilation, 15, 20–1
Basic life support, 7
  active chest compression/decompression, 22
  adults, 9–18
  children and infants, 83–90
    newborn babies, 108–11
  choking, 17–20, 89–90
  compression to breath ratio, 18
    children and babies, 86, 88, 110
  hypothermia, 59
  impact of time to implementation, 120
  near drowning, 57–8
  newborn babies, 108–11
  poisoning, 61
  precordial thump, 19–20
  risks to rescuer, 20–1
  training, 8, 124, 129–31
  trauma cases, 66